Herbal Remedies

for everyday living

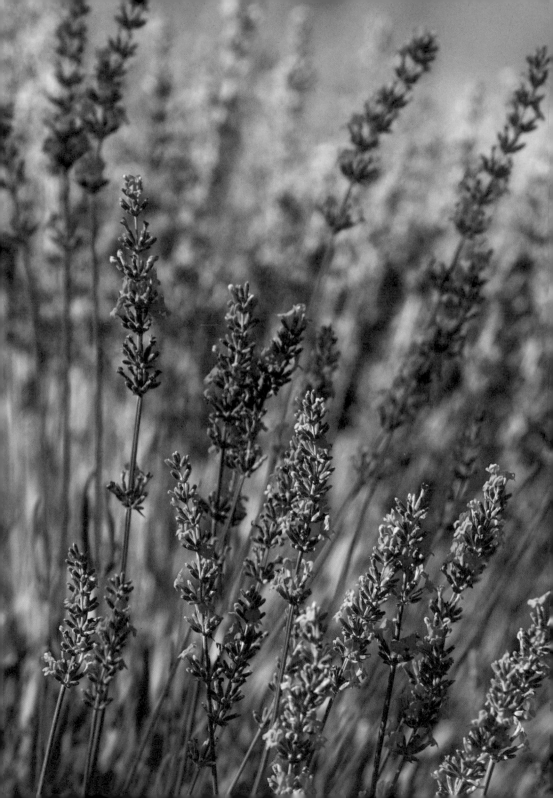

Herbal Remedies

for everyday living

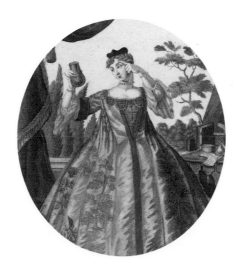

Anne McIntyre

An Hachette UK Company
www.hachette.co.uk

This edition published in 2015 by Bounty Books,
a division of Octopus Publishing Group Ltd
Carmelite House
50 Victoria Embankment
London, EC4Y 0DZ
www.octopusbooks.co.uk

ISBN: ISBN 978-0-7537-2974-8

A CIP catalogue record for this book is available from the
British Library

Printed and bound in China

10 9 8 7 6 5 4 3 2

Publisher's note: *Herbal remedies should be used with care.
Many herbs are unsuitable for use with particular medical
conditions. Always refer to the safety warnings before using
any of the herbs. While the advice and information in this
book is believed to be accurate, neither the author nor the
publisher can accept any legal responsibility for any injury
sustained whilst following any of the suggestions herein.*

CONTENTS

INTRODUCTION

This book provides a practical, accessible reference guide to the use of 140 common herbs in the modern practice of Western herbal medicine, and by doing so highlights the great contribution herbs can make to modern medical care. There is an emphasis on how herbs are used most effectively when they are prescribed after the taking of a full case history, with the intention of aiding innate homeostatic mechanisms while addressing the underlying problems that give rise to health problems, including diet and lifestyle.

ANCIENT AND MODERN MEDICINE

A conventional medical view might take some exception to aspects of herbal philosophy and approach to treatment that may follow some rather unorthodox lines. There may not be much scientific justification for, for example, the use of 'alterative' or cleansing herbs to clear the body of toxins, or cooling herbs to clear 'accumulated heat', but they are integral to the philosophies of ancient and respected systems, such as Chinese, Tibetan and Ayurvedic medicine, that have survived almost intact for at least 5,000 years.

We can trace the link between human life and healing herbs back to Neanderthal man 60,000 years ago, when herbs including Horsetail, Yarrow and Ephedra were used. With the vast network of communication that has developed in recent decades has come a wealth of information and wisdom from far and wide that has engendered a considerable merging of herbal traditions. This means that herbalists today have the advantage of drawing on a number of therapeutic systems and philosophies, as well as access to the herbs themselves from most corners of the globe.

Some therapeutic traditions – such as Chinese, Ayurvedic, Unani Tibb and Tibetan medicine – are based on systems of healing that have remained almost intact through thousands of years and still form the primary healthcare system for a significant proportion of the population in those countries. Many Western herbalists now study those traditions and incorporate their ancient practices into their own diagnosis and treatments.

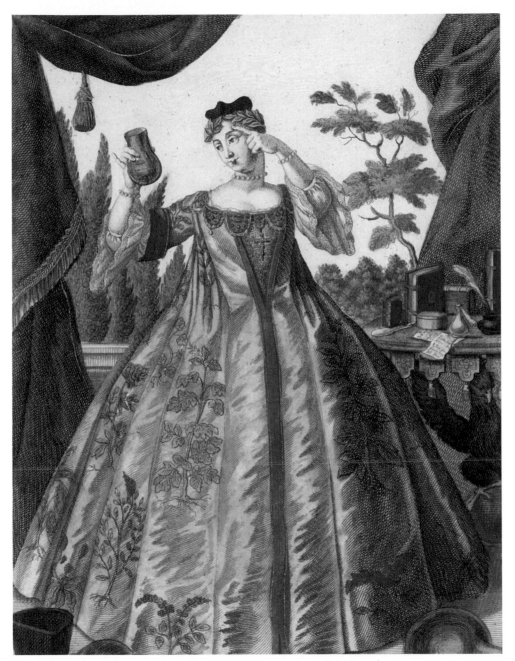

This 18th century German engraving depicts a female herbalist at work.

Other age-old systems of herbal healing, particularly in the Western world, have been largely broken and replaced by modern drugs and conventional medicine. Currently, the popularity of herbal medicine has inspired a re-evaluation of global medical roots, with their rich sources of effective medicines that certainly have a place in modern medical practice. Herbs such as Garlic, Ginkgo, Ginseng, Echinacea and St John's wort have proved themselves to the world, almost becoming household names in the process, and are even sometimes recommended by doctors.

In recent decades the scientific world has identified specific constituents of herbs and their properties and interactions. Modern studies into the efficacy of herbs and randomized controlled trials have proven that herbs can be effective medicines, and this research vindicates the ancient use of such plants that goes back thousands of years.

PRACTICAL GUIDANCE

The hedgerows, our gardens and the shelves of health-food stores and pharmacies are lined with dazzling arrays of herbs that can be overwhelming to many who feel they lack the necessary knowledge to choose those appropriate to their needs with confidence. The media presentation of herbs has shifted from extolling the virtues of herbs and their 'miraculous cures', declaring that everything natural had to be safe and free from the side effects of modern drugs, to the opposite view, which perhaps makes more exciting reading, alarming the public that herbs have potential side effects and may even be dangerous. Without sufficient real evidence it is easy for lay people and professionals to be susceptible to such hype, but with more information it is possible to have a more realistic view.

This book will serve all those using herbs for themselves, their friends and family or their patients, who wish to learn more about the safe and effective use of herbal medicines and navigate themselves through questions regarding dosage, interactions and contraindications so that they can use herbs with the confidence they deserve. The format of the ailments section follows a body-system approach, including the main systems affected by common illness, and the health problems covered in the text are those that are frequently encountered by professional herbalists.

Please note that, in describing the herbal treatment of many common ailments, this book is not intended to replace proper medical care, which may require the greater knowledge and expertise of the professional medical herbalist or mainstream healthcare practitioner.

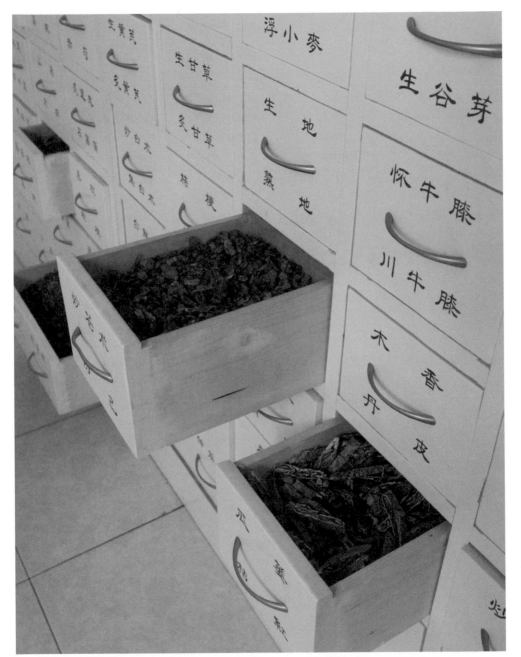

Traditional Chinese herbal treatment has been shown to be effective in treating eczema.

PART I:
HERBAL BASICS

How do herbs work on the human organism? Much of their medicinal action can be classified according to a plant's therapeutic constituents. However, plants work synergistically – the whole being more than the sum of the parts – and this has been less well studied. As a result, many herbalists are happy to evaluate the healing potential of plants according to both modern scientific findings and more holistic philosophies of energy medicine.

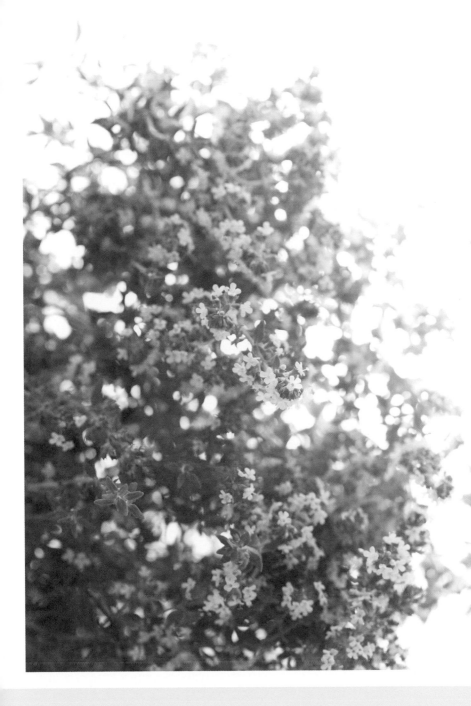

THE CHEMISTRY OF HERBS

For thousands of years, until the last 200 years or so, plants provided the sole source of medicines, and many familiar medicines of the 21st century have been derived directly or indirectly from herbs. Despite this, there are still those who persist in the view that the value of herbs is unproven scientifically.

At the same time, the value and popularity of herbs as medicines in recent years has prompted more research into the action of plant components. Alongside this has come a re-emergence in popularity of ancient systems of medicine, with their 'holistic' philosophies, as well as more modern systems of healing using plants, such as aromatherapy. This has occurred amid a milieu of natural healing that has challenged modern medicine to the point that now many people are aware that valid choices exist before a patient embarks on a course of treatment.

WHOLE-PLANT MEDICINES

To stand up to scrutiny in a modern scientific world, herbalists now have to provide evidence of the efficacy and safety of therapeutic herbs they use and apply the tools of the scientific world – biochemistry and pharmacology – to their task. While herbalists advocate the use of whole-plant medicines, their enquiry necessitates that, for study and evaluation purposes, ingredients are singled out and their actions are ascertained. Such research enables quality testing and efficient extraction methods, and provides pointers to potential side effects and herb–drug interactions. Once this is accomplished, it does not, however, tell the whole story, and the knowledge gained from such study still needs to be incorporated into a more overall view of the whole plant.

It has long been held that a herb is more than the sum of its parts, and despite investigations into what are seen as the active ingredients in a given plant, there are other 'lesser' constituents that have an equally important role to play therapeutically. They are essential in determining how effective the primary healing agents will be by rendering the body more or less receptive to their powers. Some of these 'synergistic' substances will make the active constituents more easily assimilated and readily available in the body, while others will buffer the action of other potent plant chemicals, thus preventing the risk of side effects. It is the natural combination of both types of substance that determines the healing power and safety of any herbal medicine.

Before the development of modern scientific methods for isolating active constituents, whole-plant medicines were used. As science progressed, many of these constituents were able to be synthesized, perhaps in the assumption that synthetic compounds were similar to those derived from the plant world and, as such, would be assimilated just as easily by the body. Herbs became more or less redundant. However, chemical analysis of medicinal plants has demonstrated that there is a similarity in the molecular structure of components of plants that makes the foods we eat and herbs used as medicines easily assimilated. The isolation and synthesis of potent active ingredients can produce an array of side effects. Plant-derived drugs such as morphine, digoxin, ephedrine and atropine clearly need to be used with great caution.

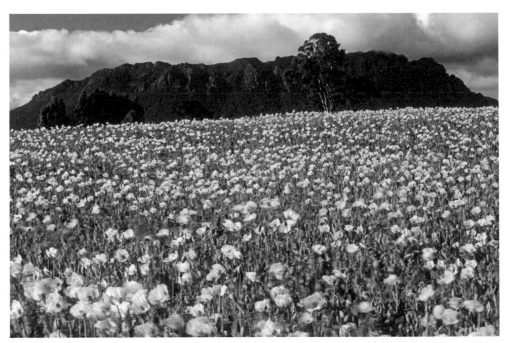

Opium poppies in Tasmania, Australia; some fifty per cent of the world's crop used in medicine is grown here.

CONSTITUENTS OF HERBAL MEDICINES

Through photosynthesis, plants manufacture carbohydrates and give off oxygen, and in this process they create metabolic pathways that provide building blocks for the production of a vast array of compounds.

In medicinal plants these include minerals, vitamins and trace elements, and a vast assortment of substances known to have specific therapeutic actions in the body. The more widely known of these follow.

PHENOLS

Phenols are a large class of secondary plant compounds. They are aromatic alcohols and the building blocks of many plant components, and generally have antiseptic, antibacterial and anthelmintic actions. One simple phenolic compound is salicylic acid, which forms glycosides found in Willow and Meadowsweet. It has antiseptic, painkilling and anti-inflammatory properties and forms the basis of aspirin.

Among other compounds are the hydroxycinnamic acids including caffeic, ferulic and sinapic acids. These form the basis of phenolic esters, coumarins, glycosides and lignans, as well as cynarin and curcumin, the main component of Turmeric, famous as an anti-inflammatory agent which also lowers blood pressure and protects the liver.

COUMARINS

These occur widely in plants, including Black cohosh, Wild oats, Angelica and Horse chestnut, and are generally antimicrobial and antifungal. They generally occur as glycosides, for example aescin in Horse chestnut. Dicoumarol, originally derived from Sweet clover (Melilotus officinalis), is used as a strong anticlotting agent in the form of warfarin in allopathic medicine.

Furanocoumarins include angelican and archangelican from Angelica root, which are antispasmodic. These need to be used cautiously, as they can cause photosensitivity, increasing the effect of sunlight on the skin, but could be used therapeutically for vitiligo and psoriasis.

ANTHRAQUINONES

These glycosides are found in Senna, and Yellow dock, and pass unaltered through the stomach and small intestine and are converted to their active form by micro-organisms. They stimulate peristalsis and inhibit water reabsorption in the large intestine, producing a laxative effect.

TANNINS

These occur widely in nature, often as glycosides, and represent the largest group of polyphenols. Tannins are the main therapeutic constituents in Witch hazel, Agrimony, Raspberry leaf and Meadowsweet. Their main therapeutic action is astringent. On the skin or in the delicate linings of the mouth and respiratory, digestive, urinary and reproductive systems, tannins can separate bacteria that threaten to invade from their source of nutrition. They occur either as hydrolysable or condensed tannins. The former protect the skin and mucosa from irritation and reduce swelling and inflammation. The latter include oligomeric procyanidins, known for their antioxidant and cardiovascular properties.

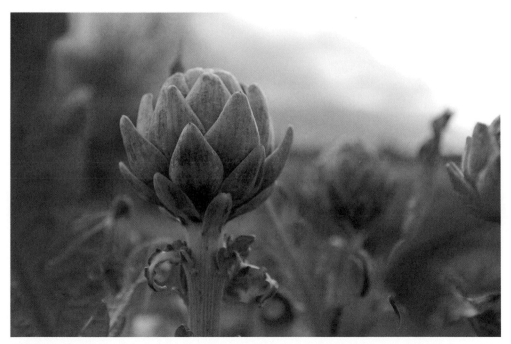

Globe artichoke is a rich source of cynarin, a phenolic compound that supports the liver and can lower cholesterol.

FLAVONOIDS

Flavonoids occur widely in nature and impart a yellow, orange and red colour to fruits and flowers. Their antioxidant action makes them an important part of our diet, having a beneficial effect on the heart and circulation, strengthening and healing blood vessel walls and enhancing resilience to stress. They act synergistically with ascorbic acid to enhance the body's ability to metabolize it. They are anti-inflammatory, antitumour, antiviral and hypotensive. Herbs rich in flavonoids such as kaempferol, myricitin and quercitrin, protect against cardiovascular disease and treat vascular problems like bruising, piles and nosebleeds.

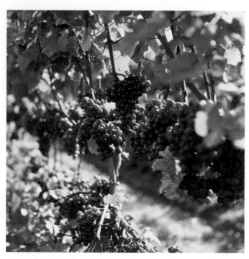

Grape seeds are good for cardiovascular health and the red skin included phenols and flavonoids.

TERPENES

Terpenes occur in a variety of forms, including monoterpenes, sesquiterpenes and triterpenes.

Monoterpenes are the main components of volatile oils, and include bitter iridoids as in the sedative valepotriates in Valerian, hypotensive asperulsides in Cleavers and paeoniflorin in Peony, which has anti-inflammatory, febrifuge and sedative actions.

Sesquiterpenes are also found in volatile oils or as lactones, and have a bitter taste, anti-inflammatory and antimicrobial actions. Sesquiterpenes are found in Myrrh, Hops, Chamomile and Chaste tree, and sesquiterpene lactones occur in Feverfew, Yarrow, Wormwood, Globe artichoke and Elecampane.

Triterpenes have a similar structure to steroids (see below).

BITTERS

Bitters are diverse in structure, but have certain therapeutic actions in common and include mostly terpenes, flavonoids and some alkaloids. Through their effect on the bitter receptors on the tongue they promote the secretion of digestive enzymes from the stomach and intestines, the flow of bile from the liver and the release of hormones.

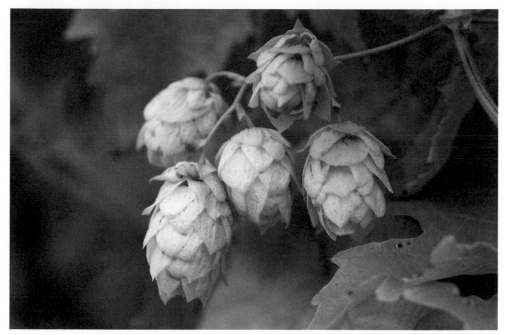

Hops are bitter, promoting the secretion of digestive enzymes, bile and certain hormones; they also have sedative properties.

Bitters are prescribed for poor appetite and digestion, gastritis, heartburn, to regulate blood sugar, relieve allergies and inflammation.

TRITERPENOIDS

Triterpenoids represent a large and diverse group that includes phytosterols, saponins, triterpenoid saponins, steroidal saponins and cardiac glycosides.

Phytosterols have been used as building blocks for making steroid drugs and may have the ability to inhibit tumour formation Phytosterols such as sitosterol and stigmasterol are vital to the formation of cell membranes and help regulate cholesterol.

Saponins are glycosides that precipitate cholesterol. Herbs containing saponins have a bitter taste and haemolytic activity. They can dissolve red blood cell walls, so should never be injected into the bloodstream. Taken orally, however, they are hardly absorbed through an intact intestine and help to promote digestion and absorption of nutrients such as calcium and silicon.

Triterpenoid saponins help regulate steroidal hormonal activity and counter the effects of stress, and often have antifungal properties. Herbs containing these properties are known as adaptogens, the most famous of which is Korean ginseng.

Steroidal saponins are used in the body as building blocks for the production of hormones secreted by the testes, ovaries and adrenal glands, and vitamin D.

Cardiac glycosides have been widely researched for their ability to increase cardiac output by affecting the force and speed of heart contractions, which is beneficial in heart failure. Herbs containing these are generally for use by practitioners only.

VOLATILE OILS

The exotic perfumes and delicious tastes of aromatic herbs are derived from volatile oils, which are complex combinations of compounds; up to 60 different chemical constituents have been identified in some oils. Categories of volatile oils include terpenoids and phenylpropanoids.

All volatile oils are antiseptic, stimulating the production of white blood cells and enhancing immunity. Many oils have antibacterial, antifungal and antiviral actions, and also anti-inflammatory and antispasmodic properties, particularly those containing sesquiterpenes. While they exert beneficial effects on the body, oils also reach the brain and nervous system and have a wide range of mento-emotional applications.

FIXED OILS

These are lipids found in all plants, especially the seeds, and contain fatty acids that are either saturated, monounsaturated or polyunsaturated.

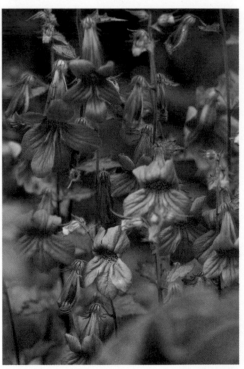

Chinese foxglove is prescribed by herbalists for its cardiac glycosides, a type of saponin that increases cardiac output.

They are vital for growth, formation of cell membranes and functioning of the immune and cardiovascular systems. Two that exist in every cell, particularly in the nervous system, known as essential fatty acids, are linoleic acid and linolenic acid, which are not able to be synthesized in the body and need to be taken in the diet. In the body, linoleic acid is converted into gamma-linolenic acid (GLA). Atopic allergies such as eczema and asthma and other immune problems are related to the lack of the enzyme responsible for this conversion in some individuals.

POLYSACCHARIDES

These sugar molecules are found widely in the plant world, for example in fructose, glucose and cellulose, and consist of chains of sugars linked to other molecules. They include mucilage, gums and fructans. Some polysaccharides, particularly beta-glucans found in, for instance, Reishi and Shiitake mushrooms, have immunostimulating properties. They activate cytokines that enhance the production of white blood cells and antibodies, and also have anti-inflammatory and antitumour actions.

MUCILAGE

This sugary, gel-like substance draws water to it to form a viscous fluid. When taken orally, mucilage coats the mucous membranes of the digestive, respiratory and genitourinary tracts, protecting them from irritation and inflammation. Herbs rich in mucilage such as Slippery elm, Marshmallow, Plantain and Coltsfoot are prescribed for their cooling and soothing properties. They relieve diarrhoea by reducing peristalsis caused by irritation of the gut lining, but can be used as laxatives, absorbing water into the bowel and bulking out the stool, as in Psyllium seeds.

FRUCTANS

These are composed of fructose and occur especially in herbs in the Compositae family as inulin, such as Globe artichoke, Goldenrod, Gentian, Codonopsis and Burdock. Inulin helps regulate blood sugar and enhances the immune system.

ALKALOIDS

The chemicals in this diverse group contain a nitrogen-bearing molecule and are pharmacologically very potent. Many of the more toxic plants contain alkaloids, such as atropine in Belladonna and morphine in the Opium poppy. Caffeine, ephedrine, quinine, strychnine, piperine, nicotine and codeine are all alkaloids with diverse actions ranging from stimulants, bronchodilators, antimicrobials and anti-inflammatories to narcotics and painkillers.

MEDICINAL ACTIONS OF HERBS

The following guide classifies herbs according to their medicinal action (see The Materia Medica, pages 46–119).

Alteratives: Barberry, Bladderwrack, Blue flag, Burdock, Cleavers, Comfrey, Dandelion, Devil's claw, Echinacea, Elderflower, Eyebright, Garlic, Golden seal, Brahmi, Holy thistle, Liquorice, Marshmallow, Nettle, Oregon grape root, Poke root, Red clover, St John's wort, Sarsaparilla

Analgesic/Anodyne: California poppy, Chamomile, Hops, Passion flower, St John's wort, Valerian, Wild lettuce

Anthelmintic: Aloe vera, Garlic, Senna, Thyme, Walnut , Wormwood

Anticatarrhal: Coltsfoot, Elder, Elecampane, Eyebright, Garlic, Goldenrod, Golden seal, Hyssop, Marshmallow, Mullein, Sage, Thyme, Yarrow

Anti-inflammatory: Chamomile, Devil's claw, Frankincense, Ginger, Liquorice, Marigold, St John's wort, Turmeric, Witch hazel

Antimicrobial: Clove, Coriander, Echinacea, Elecampane, Garlic, Liquorice, Marigold, Myrrh, Peppermint, Rosemary, Sage, St John's wort, Thyme, Wormwood

Antispasmodic: Black cohosh, Black haw, Chamomile, Cramp bark, Lime flower, Mistletoe, Motherwort, Pasque flower, Thyme, Valerian, Vervain

Astringent: Agrimony, Bayberry, Beth root, Cramp bark, Elecampane, Eyebright, Goldenrod, Ground ivy, Meadowsweet, Mullein, Myrrh, Raspberry, Rosemary, Sage, Vervain, Witch hazel leaf

Bitter: Barberry, Dandelion root, Devil's claw, Globe artichoke, Golden seal, Hops, Ho shou wu, Sweet Annie, White horehound, Wood betony, Wormwood, Yarrow

Carminative: Angelica root, Chamomile, Cinnamon, Dill, Fennel, Ginger, Hyssop, Lavender, Lemon balm, Peppermint, Rosemary

Cholagogue: Barberry, Blue flag, Gentian, Globe artichoke, Peppermint, Yellow dock

Demulcent: Chickweed, Comfrey, Fenugreek, Liquorice, Marshmallow, Mullein, Plantain, Slippery elm

Diaphoretic: Angelica root, Bayberry, Chamomile, Elderflower, Elecampane, Ginger, Goldenrod, Hyssop, Lemon balm, Lime flower, Peppermint, Pleurisy root, Prickly ash, Vervain, Yarrow

Diuretic: Buchu, Corn silk, Couch grass, Dandelion leaf and root, Globe artichoke, Goldenrod, Gravel root, Horsetail, Shatavari, Wild celery seed

Emmenagogue: Beth root, Black cohosh, Black haw, Chamomile, Chaste tree, Cramp bark, Fenugreek, Gentian, Ginger, Golden seal, Holy thistle, Marigold, Motherwort, Pasque flower, Peppermint, Raspberry, Rosemary, St John's wort, Thyme, Valerian, Vervain, Wormwood, Yarrow

Emollient: Borage, Chickweed, Coltsfoot, Comfrey, Elecampane, Fenugreek, Liquorice, Marshmallow, Mullein, Plantain, Rose petals, Slippery elm

Expectorant: Angelica root, Elecampane, Fennel, Ground ivy, Hyssop, Liquorice, Marshmallow, Mullein, Pleurisy root, Thyme, Vervain, White horehound

Febrifuge: Borage, Elderflower, Holy thistle, Hyssop, Lemon balm, Marigold, Peppermint, Plantain, Pleurisy root, Prickly ash, Raspberry, Thyme, Vervain

Hepatic: Agrimony, Aloe vera, Barberry, Blue flag, Cleavers, Dandelion, Elecampane, Fennel, Gentian, Globe artichoke, Golden seal, Hyssop, Kalamegha, Lemon balm, Motherwort, Prickly ash, Rosemary, Schisandra, Wild celery, Wild yam, Wormwood, Yarrow, Yellow dock

Laxative: Aloe vera resin, Barberry, Blue flag, Burdock, Chinese angelica, Cleavers, Dandelion leaf and root, Liquorice, Senna, Slippery elm, Yellow dock

Mucilage: Comfrey, Fenugreek, Marshmallow, Slippery elm

Pectoral: Chinese angelica, Coltsfoot, Comfrey, Elder, Elecampane, Garlic, Golden seal, Hyssop, Liquorice, Marshmallow, Mullein, Pleurisy root, Vervain, White horehound

Sedative: Black cohosh, Black haw, Bladderwrack, Chamomile, Cramp bark, Hops, Motherwort, Pasque flower, Passion flower, Red clover, St John's wort, Saw palmetto, Valerian, Wild yam

Stimulant: Bayberry, Bladderwrack, Cardamom, Chinese angelica, Cinnamon, Dandelion, Garlic, Gentian, Ginseng, Gravel root, Ground ivy, Marigold, Peppermint, Prickly ash, Rosemary, White horehound, Wild yam, Wormwood, Yarrow

Styptic: Horsetail, Marigold, Nettle, Witch hazel leaf, Yarrow

Tonic: Agrimony, Angelica, Bayberry, Beth root, Buchu, Burdock, Chamomile, Chinese angelica, Cleavers, Coltsfoot, Comfrey, Couch grass, Dandelion, Echinacea, Elecampane, Eyebright, Garlic, Gentian, Ginseng, Golden seal, Gravel root, Ground ivy, Hawthorn, Horse chestnut, Hyssop, Lemon balm, Liquorice, Marigold, Mistletoe, Motherwort, Myrrh, Nettle, Poke root, Raspberry, Red clover, Sarsaparilla, Thyme, Vervain, Wild oats, Wild yam, Wood betony, Yarrow

THE HERBAL CONSULTATION

Before you make a diagnosis, prescribe remedies and prepare herbal medicines, it is essential to understand the concepts of holism and homeostasis, and how plants can enhance the body's innate healing processes. Treating underlying causes and not simply addressing symptoms forms the basis of a herbalist's practice, and every consultation, treatment plan and herbal prescription is tailored to individual patients with the aim of bringing positive and lasting results.

HEALING THE WHOLE PERSON

Modern medical herbalism is a synthesis of ancient and modern theories and practices, and its underlying philosophy is that health is intimately connected to the harmony of body, mind and spirit, which enables a balance of natural forces within the body. In a clinical context, the herbalist will interpret any symptoms of ill health as a disturbance of this balance and consider them in the context of the patient as a whole and their lives, both inner and outer.

In addition to redressing specific imbalances, herbalists should ideally prescribe plant remedies in order to attend to the deeper causes of that imbalance, setting their treatments within a framework of life-affirming lifestyles and eating habits.

The herbalist recognizes that the human body is made up of a complex organization of tissues and cells that operate on a molecular level, and yet the human organism is so much more than this.

LIFE FORCE

Behind the physical manifestation that is the body is the existence of subtle energy, which is recognized by mythology and religion but largely denied by modern science. It is known throughout the world by different names: life force, vital force, 'qi' and 'prana'. We can neither see it nor define it, but it is there and we are animated by this living force on every level of existence – physical, emotional, mental and spiritual. Through this we have an inherent ability to regulate the functions of the body and to heal ourselves, which is

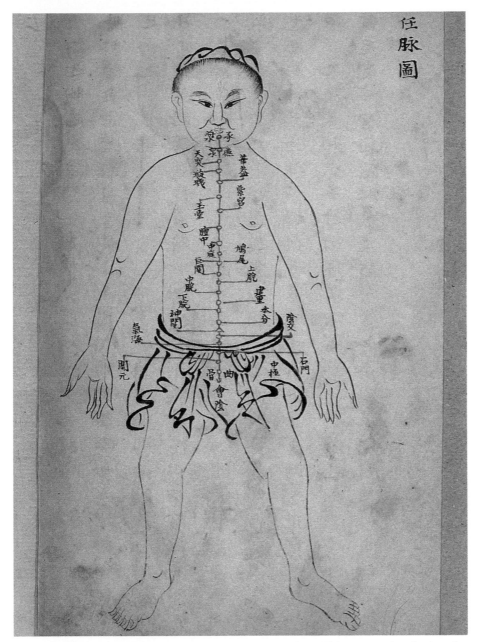

Qi, or life force, flows along energy channels, or meridians. This manuscript depicts the Conception Vessel meridian.

known in the West as homeostasis. When this life force is disturbed on any level, the health of the whole person is affected and illness results. Body, emotion, mind and spirit form one interrelated system and an imbalance in one creates disharmony in another. Symptoms of ill health in the body represent the attempt by the organism to correct the imbalance and heal itself. If these symptoms are suppressed, as they are by modern drugs, the energy of the vital force is depleted, our healing ability dwindles and finally chronic illness results. The body needs to be permitted to express its symptoms as far as possible, and any treatment should be aimed at augmenting the efforts of the vital force, to enhance its healing energy and not work against it. The task of the herbalist is to analyse a patient's presenting symptoms in this respect and to support the body's homeostatic mechanisms through the use of herbs and lifestyle guidance. A maxim of natural therapy is that medicine cannot change the workings of the body; it can only help them. One of the oldest medical teachings is 'Medicus curat, natura sanat' – 'The doctor treats, but nature heals'.

USING HERBS AS MEDICINES

Herbalists use the leaves, flowers, bark, berries, roots or seeds of medicinal plants as their therapeutic tools. By definition, a herb is any plant that has a medicinal action in the body, and this includes most fruits and vegetables. In fact, herbs act very much like foods, and many common foods are used for their medicinal actions: carrots are good for skin; oats are a great tonic for the nervous system; garlic fights infection and regulates blood pressure.

Plants absorb vital nutrients from the soil and then process and store them, providing raw materials – close in chemical composition to those that make up the human body, for growth and repair of bodily tissues – that are easily digested and assimilated. Their vitamins, minerals and trace elements are vital for health and recovery, while other medicinal substances they contain, such as tannins, volatile oils, phenols and saponins have affinities with particular tissues and systems, and act more specifically to promote homeostasis and healing.

Herbs and life force

Clearly then, herbs operate at the level of biochemical reactions in the body, but they are capable of so much more. They certainly provide us with a wealth of wonderful chemicals, but their healing power goes far beyond the physical to the realms of the vital force. When herbs work in the body, they enhance the healing action of the vital life force, and as they do this, they may also heal our hearts and our minds, for they help to restore balance and harmony to an integrated whole.

THE FIRST VISIT

Prepare for a first visit by compiling lists of present symptoms, past medical and drug history, illnesses and operations as far back as infancy. Medical reports from other health consultants, as well as blood profiles, urine analyses, allergy tests and X-ray or scan reports, can provide important information. A diary of food eaten over the previous weeks may also be helpful.

A herbalist will always enquire into mento-emotional realms and some people may find it helpful to prepare for this, since it may be challenging for them to talk about painful experiences or they may not be accustomed to talking about themselves.

INDIVIDUAL EVALUATION

The consultation begins the minute patient meets practitioner. Consciously or unconsciously, the practitioner will be assessing the patient in considerable detail. The hue and tone of the skin, the brightness of the eyes and hair, the colour of the lips, the expression on the face, the tone of voice, general appearance and dress sense all begin to tell the story. Then there is body language: the expression in the face, the level of tension in the muscles, gait and posture all convey important messages.

During the consultation the patient is given time and opportunity to describe his or her concerns in detail. Each person is evaluated as an individual by the herbalist, who records and analyses current presenting symptoms in relation to the person's complete medical history in order to understand the underlying causes and contributing factors that have made the patient seek help.

Through questioning, the practitioner will systematically go through all of the major bodily systems, and the status of his or her functions will all contribute to the analysis of the total health picture of the patient.

This will be followed by necessary and relevant physical examinations, which may include tongue, urine and pulse diagnoses, blood pressure, listening to the heart or chest, palpating the abdomen, examining the nails, eyes and skin.

TREATMENT

The treatment of most ailments begins at home. Many people are almost unwittingly using herbal medicine in common household remedies like salt gargles for sore throats, hot lemon and honey drinks for colds and catarrh, Chamomile tea for sleep, Peppermint to settle the stomach, vinegar for wasp stings and Dock leaves for nettle stings.

The more you can learn about simple remedies that could be sitting in your larder or growing in your garden or wild in the hedgerows, the more opportunity you will have to treat the first signs of acute infections and minor ailments avoiding the necessity for drugs like antibiotics, and thereby help to prevent the development of more serious disorders. Herbs used in this way make excellent preventive medicines and can enhance general well-being when taken in conjunction with a healthy diet and lifestyle.

For more chronic or serious disorders, it is advisable to consult a professional herbalist who uses herbs in the context of a holistic approach to healing, where physical symptoms are viewed in relation to other factors, including temperament, stress, social, domestic and working environment, relationships, diet, relaxation and exercise. All play a part in the emergence of an individual pattern of symptoms.

TYPES OF PATIENT

As wth patients using conventional medicines, the people who seek herbal treatments for treating their symptoms vary considerably in their needs.

Patients with chronic disorders

Most people who consult a herbalist with chronic disorders do so because either they have been treated unsuccessfully elsewhere or they are seeking a more natural alternative or complement to allopathic drugs from their doctor. Frequently, it is those whose symptoms do not fit into a classic 'disease' picture or who have symptoms for which there is little in the way of allopathy to remedy their specific situation.

Allergies such as eczema, urticaria and conjunctivitis, and hormonal, nervous and immune problems, are good examples of these. Often people come after years of coping with health problems, in which case it may take some time to return them to health. Herbal treatment can be taken alongside allopathic drugs in many instances, and a herbalist will check for any possible herb–drug interactions before prescribing.

Patients with long-term conditions

For those battling with long-term problems such as heart disease and autoimmune disease, working with a herbalist will help improve general health, energy and joie de vivre so that the patient is better able to cope with their problems.

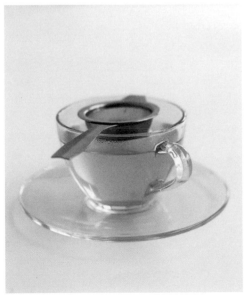

Herbal teas may be prescribed as part of dietary changes, replacing caffeinated drinks that may aggravate health problems.

Patients seeking a more holistic approach

As people are becoming more health aware in the holistic sense, they are looking to alternative or complementary health models as a first line of treatment. These people may simply feel under the weather, tired or run-down with vague symptoms that they would like to understand and resolve before they progress further.

In many cases these people may just need to have time to talk, to be heard and understood, and to activate their own self-healing mechanisms with the support of a herbal practitioner. The role of the herbalist is often that of counsellor.

SCHEDULING VISITS AND FEES

Generally, medical herbalists do not hold open surgery, as appointments tend to be lengthy and so need to be booked in advance.

A first appointment is likely to last about an hour and there may be a number of follow-up visits, each lasting 30 to 45 minutes. Many herbalists operate a sliding scale of charges for both the consultation and the herbal medicines they prescribe. They are also likely to offer reduced fees for students, pensioners, the unemployed or anyone who is experiencing hard financial times

FORMULATING A HERBAL PRESCRIPTION

Herbal prescriptions are generally tailor-made for each individual depending on their specific needs. They need to address a variety of different issues. Digestion and elimination are absolutely central to good health, and poor digestion, dysbiosis and toxicity are underlying factors in a whole range of different illnesses, including gut problems, lowered immunity, allergies, autoimmune disease, obesity and cancer.

Herbs that improve digestion and clear toxicity from the bowel are, therefore, the first considerations. Then there are herbs that need to be added for the constitutional imbalance of the system of the body affected, whether it is the nervous system in the case of anxiety and insomnia or the respiratory system in the case of bronchitis. Finally, herbs need to be included that are specific to the actual symptoms or disease, such as Frankincense for arthritis.

The method of administering herbs and the length of treatment needed by a patient will vary considerably according to the condition being treated, which herbs are used, the patient's age, build and constitution. The dosage, the herbs chosen for the prescription and the timing of administration all need to be determined. A largely built person with big bones and muscles and a comparatively sluggish metabolism will require herbs to be given in larger doses and over a longer period of time than a small-framed, lightweight person with a more sensitive body and a faster metabolism.

Dosage for adult patients can also vary according to the practitioner and which kind of herbal medicine he or she practises. A standard dose of tincture can vary from a few drops to 5 ml (1 tsp). Teas are generally taken a cupful at a time, powders are taken in doses of ¼–1 tsp and syrups may require being taken a dessertspoonful or tablespoonful at a time.

CHRONIC AND ACUTE CONDITIONS

When treating chronic conditions, generally mild herbal remedies are taken three times daily, over months at a time if necessary. It may be that the first prescription and dietary advice is intended to improve digestion and absorption, and to clear toxins from the system, which is necessary in so many cases. This will be followed up by more nourishing tonic medicines until the patient is better. Acute conditions may require stronger herbs given up to every 2 hours. For example, Echinacea and Wild indigo are taken every 2 hours to enhance immunity and combat acute infections.

APPROPRIATE ADMINISTRATION

Hot preparations are needed in fevers, colds, catarrh and problems associated with cold, such as poor circulation and menstrual cramps, while urinary problems and conditions associated with heat, such as hot flushes and acne, are better suited to cool preparations. Skin problems may improve more rapidly using herbal teas as opposed to tinctures, but tinctures may be preferable when more concentrated medicines are needed, as when treating a virulent infection.

The herbs chosen may also indicate their best method of administration. When giving teas, the aerial parts of a plant are prepared as infusions, while roots, barks and seeds are better suited to decoctions. Nourishing tonics are best taken as powders stirred into warm milk or water, and warming spices to clear catarrhal

congestion and coughs can be taken as powders mixed with honey and taken off a spoon.

Generally, herbs are taken either side of or during a meal. When using herbs to enhance appetite, digestion and absorption, they can be taken before a meal; for problems associated with heat, acidity and inflammation, they can be taken with a meal, otherwise they can be taken immediately after eating. Tinctures need to be diluted with water, otherwise they can taste unpleasant and irritate a delicate stomach.

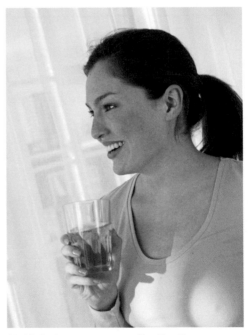

Hot infusions are more effective than tinctures for treating skin complaints, fevers, colds and catarrh.

SAFETY ISSUES

The question of possible side effects and toxicity has arisen more recently as herbs are increasingly under the scrutiny of the scientific eye. However, adverse reactions to herbal medicines seldom occur in practice, and those that do occur generally consist of mild rashes or bowel changes. A herbal practitioner would not normally expect 'healing crises', with an exacerbation of symptoms before they start to recede.

There are two main sources of information about the efficacy and safety of herbal medicines: ancient folklore and modern science. The empirical evidence gathered by herbalists over thousands of years, which is now being increasingly justified by scientific research, means that patients may be assured that their herbal prescriptions are based on reliable foundations. Many herbs form the basis of modern orthodox medicines and it may be surprising to learn that the pharmaceutical industry harvests huge plantations of herbs for use in the production of drugs each year. It also grows herbs for further research activities.

WHOLE-PLANT MEDICINES

It is the herbalist's view that the use of whole-plant medicines as opposed to isolated active ingredients helps to prevent adverse side effects.

The many types of substances in medicinal plants work synergistically together and probably all have important roles to play in the healing process. The primary healing agents are the active constituents that were isolated by the early chemists and developed into modern drugs, but the importance of the other, apparently secondary, constituents should not be ignored, as they are vital for determining the efficacy of the primary healing agents.

Some secondary synergistic substances make the active constituents more easily assimilated and available in the body, while others will buffer the action of other potent plant chemicals, preventing possible side effects from developing. It is largely the combination of both types of substance occurring in the whole plant that determines the potential potency and safety of herbal medicine.

POTENTIAL ADVERSE REACTIONS

Having said this, with the huge range of biochemical constituents that occur in herbs, it is possible that, though generally safe, some could potentially cause allergic reactions and idiosyncratic responses in the same way that foods do. Most of these can be avoided by herbalists who are generally familiar with the chemistry of herbs they are prescribing and who are in the habit of prescribing herbs that are formulated to suit the very specific needs of the patient in appropriate doses only after taking a detailed case history.

Certain people are more likely to have hypersensitive reactions to herbs than others, particularly those who already have a history of food allergy or intolerance, or chemical sensitivity. This is more likely to be the case if they suffer from digestive problems, and specifically from imbalances in the intestinal flora, intestinal dysbiosis and leaky gut syndrome, all of which also happen to lend themselves very well to treatment using herbal remedies.

Reputable sources
The risk of adulteration of herbs supplied to herbalists is one that is obviously a concern. Adverse effects have occurred on occasions owing to adulteration with toxic herbs as well as bad labelling. When buying herbs it is vital that the sources of herbs are known to be reputable and preferably organic, as adverse reactions to pesticides and preservatives are hard to quantify and could be confused with reactions to a plant itself. Indian and Chinese herbs are considered more of a safety problem than European herbs, although the use of pesticides in Eastern Europe has also attracted negative attention.

HERB–DRUG INTERACTIONS

This is a relatively new science, and very few herb–drug interactions have been recorded. Available information on the subject (much of which may be speculative rather than empirical) is growing all the time. Although herbs have been taken for thousands of years, they have been used in combination with nutritional supplements and allopathic drugs on a widespread basis for only approximately the last 30 years.

The concern is not so much that the reaction between a herb and a drug is toxic, rather that it is possible that certain herbs can affect the bioavailability of drugs and nutrients, and cause an increase or decrease in levels of drugs in the blood. This is an especially important consideration for the herbal prescriber if patients are taking specific doses of powerful drugs, such as cardiac medication and anticlotting agents or drugs given prior to surgery.

THE HERBAL PHARMACY

There are many ways to prepare beneficial herbal remedies so that they will be absorbed by the body and exert their effects. Depending on the condition being treated and the health or age of the patient, a herbalist might choose to prescribe a tea, a syrup, or an ointment to apply to the skin. Here are step-by-step instructions for preparing the most common remedies.

PREPARING HERBS

Herbs can be prepared as medicines in a variety of ways. Internal preparations such as infusions, decoctions, tinctures, syrups, honeys and tablets and capsules are swallowed so that they pass through the digestive tract and into the bloodstream. Many people are unconsciously taking remedies in their food on a daily basis, for not only do all the culinary herbs and spices add flavour to our diet but at the same time they contain volatile oils, which have digestive and antimicrobial effects among many other benefits. As the foods are absorbed from the digestive tract, so the therapeutic constituents of the herbs enter the bloodstream and then circulate round the body.

When used externally, herbs can be applied to the skin or used in herbal baths, compresses and poultices. Once in contact with the skin they are absorbed into tiny capillaries under the surface and then circulated around the body. The conjunctiva of the eye also absorbs herbal preparations. Inhalations are another very good therapeutic pathway and a main one that is utilized by aromatherapists. By inhalation into the nose, which is lined with nerve endings, the messages from the herbs are carried directly to the brain and to the lungs, where they are absorbed with oxygen into the bloodstream and circulated throughout the body.

INFUSIONS

Herbal teas, often known as infusions, are simple water-based preparations that extract the medicinal properties of herbs, used either fresh or dried. They can be drunk as teas or used externally as skin washes, eyebaths, compresses and douches, or added to baths or sitz baths.

Infusions are prepared like a normal cup of tea using the soft parts of plants, leaves, stems and flowers. Generally, infusions are best drunk when still hot, especially when treating fevers, colds and catarrh, but need to be taken lukewarm to cool for problems of the urinary tract. If necessary, they can be covered and stored in the refrigerator for up to 2 days. Some herbs need to be prepared as cold infusions, as their therapeutic components are likely to be destroyed by high temperatures. These include herbs that have a high proportion of mucilage, such as Marshmallow and Comfrey leaf. They are prepared in the same way but using cold water and left to infuse for 10–12 hours.

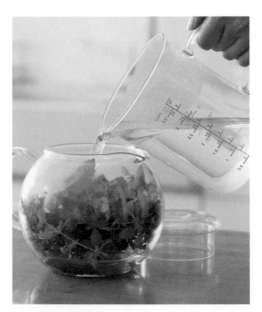
Making an infusion

To make an infusion

1 Take 50 g (2 oz) fresh herb per 600 ml (1 pint) water or 2 teaspoons of herb per cupful of water. Halve the amount of herbs if they are being used dried. Place the herbs in a warmed teapot and pour on boiling water.

2 Cover to prevent oils escaping into the atmosphere. Leave to infuse for 10–15 minutes and strain before drinking.

Dosage

Infusions are taken by the cupful three to six times a day, depending on whether the ailment being treated is chronic or acute. It may come as a surprise to some who are used to the delightful taste of culinary herbs such as Basil and Rosemary that many herbs are found by our pampered palates to taste strange, often even unpleasant. Although the bitters in some herbs need to be tasted to be effective, the bitter taste is generally not something we relish. However, it is possible to combine several herbs together in an infusion so that aromatic, pleasant-tasting herbs such as Peppermint, Fennel, Lemon balm and Lavender can disguise less-palatable herbs while not reducing their effect. Liquorice and Aniseed also make excellent herbs for flavouring. Infusions can be sweetened with honey if necessary.

TINCTURES

Tinctures are concentrated extracts of herbs made with a mixture of water and alcohol, which acts to extract the constituents of the plants and also as a preservative.

According to herbal pharmacopoeias there is a correct ratio of water and alcohol to plant matter for each herb, depending on the constituents that need extracting. This can range from 25 per cent alcohol for simple glycosides and tannins to 90 per cent for resins and gums such as those in Marigold flowers. Herbs can be used in a ratio of one part fresh herbs to two parts liquid, or one part dried herbs to five parts liquid. As an example, to make 1 litre (1¾ pints) Chamomile tincture, use 200 g (7 oz) dried flowers and 1 litre (1¾ pints) fluid. Chamomile requires a 45 per cent alcohol solution, so neat brandy or vodka would be perfectly adequate. If you have 100 per cent alcohol, use 450 ml (¾ pint) alcohol to 550 ml (18 fl oz) water.

Vinegar- and glycerol-based tinctures

Tinctures can also be prepared using neat cider vinegar, as the acetic acid acts as a solvent and preservative. Raspberry vinegar, for example, is a traditional remedy for coughs and sore throats. Glycerol-based tinctures have a sweet, syrup-like taste that makes them a good medium for children's medicines. Pour 80 per cent of glycerol and 20 per cent of water over the herbs in the same proportion of herb to liquid as for alcohol tinctures (see above). Peppermint, Lemon balm, Lavender, Rose, Holy basil, Elderflower and Mint are well suited to this method.

To make a tincture

1 Place the chopped herb in a large, clean jar and pour the water and alcohol mixture over it so that the plant is immersed. Place an airtight lid on the jar and leave it to macerate away from direct sunlight for no less than two weeks, shaking the jar well about once a day.

2 Once the tincture has macerated, use a press such as a wine press to extract as much of the fluid as possible. Alternatively, squeeze it through muslin, which is much harder work but possible. Discard the herbs, then transfer the tincture to a clean, dark, lidded bottle, label with the name of the herb and date and store in a cool, dark place.

Dosage

Because they are concentrated, only small amounts of tincture need to be taken at regular intervals through the day. The dose will vary from 5–10 drops to 1 teaspoon, taken in a little warm water, fruit juice or herbal tea, three–six times daily, depending on whether the condition is chronic or acute. Tinctures can also be added to bath water, mixed with water for compresses, mouthwashes or gargles, or stirred into a base to make ointments or creams.

Tinctures require more preparation time, but they have several advantages. They are easy to store, do not deteriorate in cold or damp conditions, take up relatively little storage space, are easy to carry around and keep almost indefinitely, although they are best taken within two years.

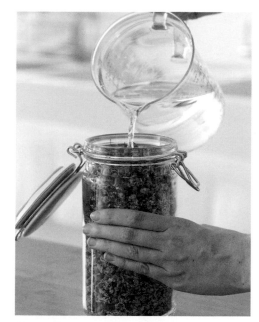

Maceration

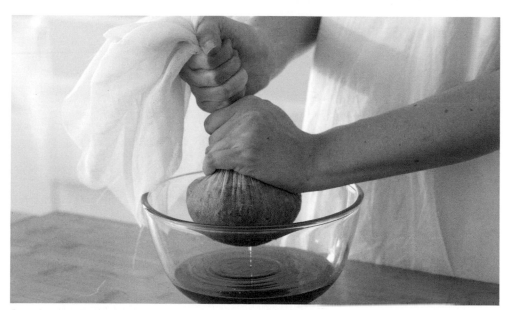

Pressing to remove fluid

SYRUPS

This type of herbal remedy is designed to make herbal preparations more palatable. Bitter herbs such as Dandelion, Burdock, Rosemary, White horehound, Yellow dock, Vervain and Motherwort are particularly suited to this method when these herbs are being prescribed for children.

Expectorant herbs for coughs, asthma and chest infections including Thyme, Hyssop, Elecampane, White horehound, Elderberry, Coltsfoot and Mullein are are often prepared as syrups, particularly when honey is included in the ingredients. Syrups can also be added to other herbal preparations to mask their more unpleasant tastes. These remedies will keep for up to two years.

To make a syrup

1 Make an infusion using 25 g (1 oz) dried herb to 600 ml (1 pint) boiling water. Double the amount of herbs if they are being used fresh. Leave to macerate in water for six to eight hours. Strain the liquid, press as much residual water from the herb before discarding it and measure how much fluid is left.

2 Pour the infusion into a saucepan and bring to the boil. Cover and simmer over a low heat until the liquid is reduced by half, which may take several hours.

3 Add 400 g (13 oz) sugar or 350 ml (12 fl oz) honey (or other sweetener of your choice) and bring to the boil until the sugar has dissolved.

4 Pour into a sterilized bottle and leave to cool. If desired, add 5 per cent of the same tincture to preserve the syrup for longer. Label the bottle clearly and store in a cool, dark place.

Dosage
Generally, 1–2 dessertspoonfuls should be taken three to four times a day for chronic problems and every two hours in acute cases.

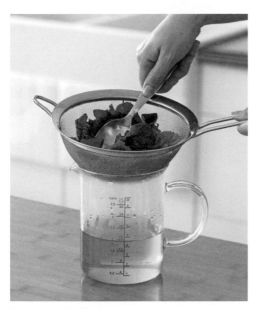

Straining the liquid

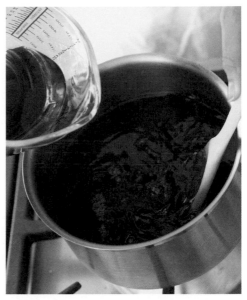

Reducing the liquid

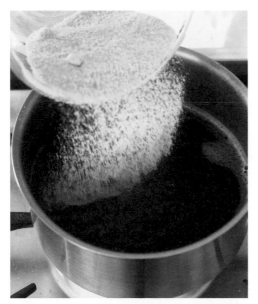

Adding sweetener

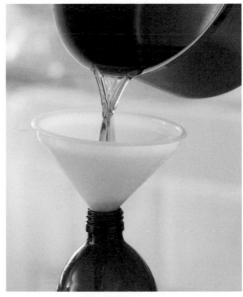

Bottling

HONEYS

Honey has been used for healing for thousands of years. It is hydroscopic, which means that it absorbs the water-soluble constituents and volatile oils of the plant. Honey has antibacterial, expectorant and healing properties, so herbal honeys can be used to treat sore throats, coughs, chest infections and asthma, and can also be used externally to heal or soothe skin problems such as cuts and grazes, burns and varicose ulcers. Honey makes an excellent medium for antimicrobial herbs such as Garlic, Thyme, Hyssop and Rosemary.

Honey is also highly nutritive, rich in easily digestible sugars and energy giving, and it enhances the immune system. It contains pollen, which is rich in protein, vitamins, minerals and fatty acids and helpful in the treatment of allergies and asthma, and propolis, which is a powerful antimicrobial. Thyme honey from Greece is renowned for its health-giving properties, as is Manuka honey from New Zealand, which is often used as an antibacterial.

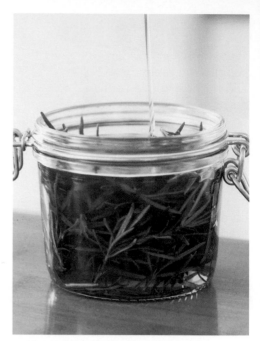

Adding honey to the herb

To make a honey

Place your chosen herbs, coarsely chopped or bruised, in a clean, sterilized jar, cover with honey and stir well. Seal with an airtight lid, label clearly and leave to macerate for at least 4 weeks but preferably several months. Store in a cool, dark place or in the refrigerator.

Dosage

Take 1 tablespoon of herbal honey in a little hot water or simply off the spoon. Do not give to children under the age of 1 due to the risk of botulinus.

Other uses for honey

You can also simply give freshly chopped herbs in a teaspoon of honey. Sweets and throat lozenges can be made by rolling powdered herbs in honey to make a paste that can be rolled into balls and then again in the powder to prevent stickiness for handling and storing. Store in a tightly fitting tin.

TABLETS AND CAPSULES

Many herbs are available from herbal suppliers in tablet or capsule form and this is a convenient way to take herbs, but it bypasses the taste buds on the tongue, which may reduce the therapeutic effects in some cases.

However, only standard preparations will be available as commercial pills, so should you require a specific combination of herbs they can be made up in gelatin capsules.

Capsules can be filled with mixtures of the appropriate herbs using a capsule maker.

To make capsules
Fill a capsule maker with open capsules, cover them with your chosen combination of powdered herbs and make sure each capsule is packed tightly. Add the capsule lids and then remove the capsules from the maker. Place in a clearly labelled container with an airtight lid and store in a cool, dark place.

Dosage
Two main sizes of capsule are used by medical herbalists: size 0, which holds 0.35 gm powder, and size 00, which holds about 0.5 gm; 1–2 size 0 capsules can be taken once daily and 1 size 00 capsule 3 times daily.

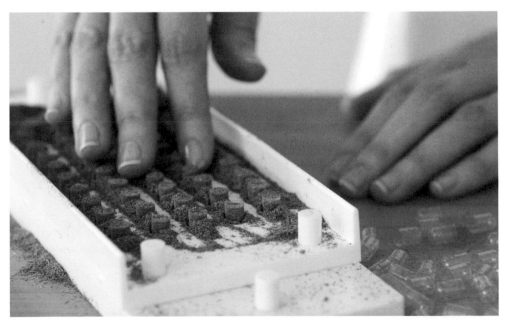

Using a capsule maker

COMPRESSES

A clean cloth or flannel can be soaked in either a hot or cold infusion, a decoction, a dilute tincture, or water with a few drops of diluted essential oil, then wrung out and applied to the affected part. This can help relieve symptoms such as headaches, abdominal colic, backache, boils and painful joints. The treatment needs to repeated several times for good effect.

LINIMENTS

A rubbing oil or liniment consists of extracts of herbs in an oil or tincture, or a mixture of both. The oils can be infused oils or essential oils diluted in a base such as sesame oil. They are used in massage to relax or stimulate muscles and ligaments or to soothe away pain from inflammation or injury. They are intended to be absorbed by the skin to reach the affected part and so they often contain a stimulating essential oil such as Ginger or Black pepper and are therefore not suitable for use on delicate baby skins.

OINTMENTS AND CREAMS

Ointments and creams can be applied to the skin not only for treatment of skin problems but also for the treatment of less superficial ailments, such as inflamed joints and headaches. Any fresh or dried herb can be made into an ointment using the recipe below.

Creams can be made easily by stirring tinctures, decoctions or a few drops of essential oil into a cream base such as aqueous cream. Many types of eczema can be effectively treated, for example, by mixing two to three drops of Chamomile oil (*Chamomilla Recutita*) into 50 g (2 oz) of any base cream that can be purchased from most herbal suppliers.

To make an ointment

1 Melt 50 g (2 oz) beeswax with 450 ml (¾ pint) olive oil in a Pyrex bowl over a saucepan of boiling water, or a double boiler.
Add as much herb as possible. Leave to macerate for a few hours over a low heat.

2 Spoon the macerated herbs into a piece of muslin placed over a jug. Allow the liquid to strain through the fabric.

3 Squeeze the muslin to press out as much of the mixture as possible and discard the herb.

4 While warm, pour into clean ointment jars to solidify quickly. Seal with an airtight lid, label and store in a cool, dark place.

Apply ointments and creams to the affected areas two to three times daily in chronic conditions, or more frequently if necessary in acute problems.

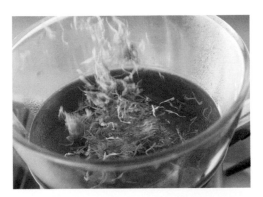

Maceration

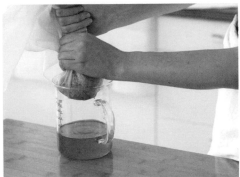

Pressing to remove

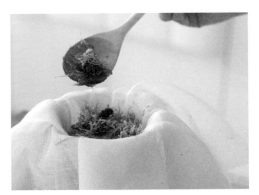

Spooning into muslin

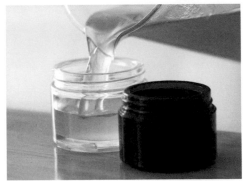

Bottling

POULTICES

These are similar to compresses but involve using the herb itself rather than an extract of the herb. Some herbs can be applied directly to the skin, such as Comfrey. They need to be softened first by removing any hard stalks or ribs and immersing them briefly in hot water to prevent any discomfort to the skin. Once applied, they can be secured in place by a light bandage and left overnight.

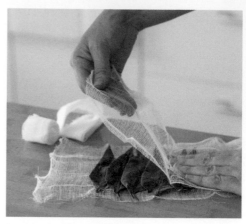

Laying the herbs in gauze

To make a poultice

1 Place the fresh or dried herb between two pieces of gauze. If you use fresh leaves, stems or roots, they need to be bruised before being applied. If the herbs are dry, add a little hot water to powdered or finely chopped herbs to make a paste.

2 Use a light cotton bandage to bind the gauze poultice to the affected part and keep it warm with a hot water bottle. Replace after 4 hours and apply about 3 times daily.

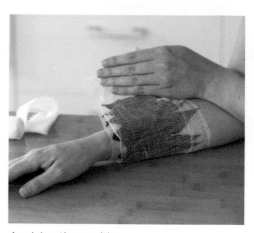

Applying the poultice

DECOCTIONS

The hard, woody parts of plants have tough cell walls that require greater heat to break them down before they will release their constituents into the water. Bark, seeds, roots, rhizomes and nuts all need to be prepared as decoctions. Use the same proportion of herbs to water as you do when preparing an infusion, but just add a little more water to make up for losses during boiling.

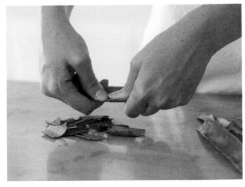
Breaking down woody parts

To make a decoction

1 Break the herb up into small pieces, crush with a pestle and mortar or smash with a hammer if very hard.

2 Place the herbs in a stainless steel or enamel saucepan and cover with cold water. Bring to the boil, then reduce the heat, cover and simmer for 10–15 minutes.

3 Strain and drink in the same way as an infusion.

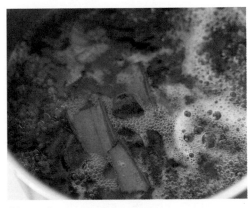
Simmering

Dosage
As for infusions.

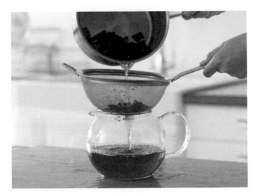
Straining

OILS

Essential oils need to be used with care, especially with children and babies. They can be used diluted in a base oil such as sesame oil (1–2 drops of essential oil per 5 ml/1 teaspoon of base oil) for massage and use in the bath. They can also be used neat in burners to permeate the atmosphere or in inhalations for a variety of symptoms such as colds, catarrh, coughs, insomnia and anxiety.

While essential oils are extracted from aromatic plants professionally by steam distillation, infused oils can easily be prepared at home. Place finely chopped, preferably fresh herbs in a jar with a tight-fitting lid, cover them with an oil such as almond, coconut, olive or sesame, pouring it up to the top of the jar, and then stir well. Add the lid, label the jar with the name of the herb and the date, then place the jar on a sunny windowsill to macerate for approximately four to eight weeks. Be aware that if there is any moisture on the plant or jar, or if it is left for longer than the specified time, the oil may go mouldy.

The oil gradually takes up the plant constituents; you can see this in action with St John's wort. In minutes the oil will turn deep red. After two weeks, filter the oil through muslin, squeezing to extract it. Store in a clean, dark, labelled bottle with an airtight lid in a cool, dark place.

HERBAL BATHS

A fragrant hot bath makes a very pleasant and simple way to take herbs. There are various ways of adding herbs to bath water: you can dilute essential oils (1 drop of essential oil per 5 ml of base oil such as sesame oil) and add them into the bathwater; hang a muslin bag containing fresh or dried aromatic herbs under the hot tap as you draw the bath; or pour 600 ml (1 pint) of strong herbal infusion into the water. Soak in the bath for 10–20 minutes.

When herbs are used in this way, the essential oils from the plants are taken in via the pores of the skin, which are opened up by the warmth of the water. The oils are also carried on the steam, which is simultaneously inhaled via nose and mouth into the lungs and from there into the bloodstream. From the nose, messages are carried from the oils via nerve pathways to the brain. Herbal medicines are assimilated quickly and directly in this way, bypassing the lengthy process of digestion necessary when herbs are taken by mouth. They are particularly useful for relaxing and soothing the nervous system and for easing mental and emotional strain.

Lavender, Lemon balm, Holy basil, Rose and Chamomile are not only wonderfully fragrant but also relaxing, calming tension and anxiety and helping to ensure restful sleep.

Chamomile is excellent for fractious children, particularly when they are unwell, for not only does it possess antimicrobial properties but it also helps induce sleep – nature's best way to ward off infection and enable self-healing. Rosemary baths, while also relaxing, have a stimulating edge, as they enhance blood flow to the head and enable greater alertness and concentration.

Herbal sitz baths can be very useful for soothing the pain and irritation of cystitis, vaginal infections or haemorrhoids. Simply fill a large, shallow bowl with about 1 litre (1¾ pints) of strained, strong infusion, enough to reach the necessary areas, sit in it and relax for 10–15 minutes.

Hand and foot baths

Mustard foot baths were historically used for all afflictions of cold and damp climates, from colds and flu to poor circulation and arthritis. The ancient tradition of hand and foot baths was popularized by the famous French herbalist Maurice Mességué. He recommends foot baths for 8 minutes in the evening and hand baths for 8 minutes in the morning. The hands and feet are, according to Mességué, highly sensitive areas of the skin, rich in nerve endings, and despite some thickening of the skin from use, the constituents pass easily from the skin into the body. To try this, add 1 tablespoon of mustard powder to a bowl of warm water and sit with your feet in it for 8 minutes.

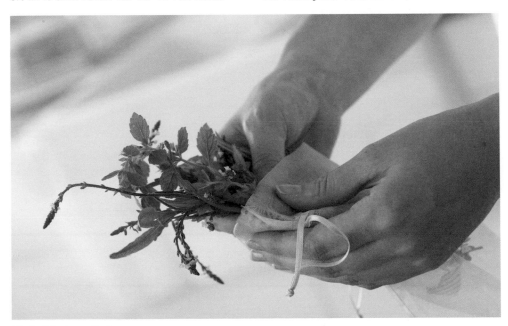

Herb-filled muslin bag

PART II:
THE MATERIA MEDICA

A material medica is a compendium of medicinal herbs used for their therapeutic effects, and traditionally describes each herb's medicinal actions. What follows is a comprehensive directory of the 140 herbs most commonly used by modern Western herbalists, organized alphabetically by Latin name. Each entry includes the common name, family, parts used, and the principle actions of the plant. It then lists the herb's indications for use in treatment according to the systems of the body. This makes for easy cross-reference to the 'Treating common ailments' section of the book so that you can be informed about the herbs that you choose. All of the herbs in the following pages are easily available from most herbal suppliers, and because this book is intended for use by lay people as well as students and practitioners of herbal medicine, none of them is a 'Schedule 3' herb, that is herbs whose dosage is restricted by law due to the presence of powerful constituents, often alkaloids, that require caution in their use.

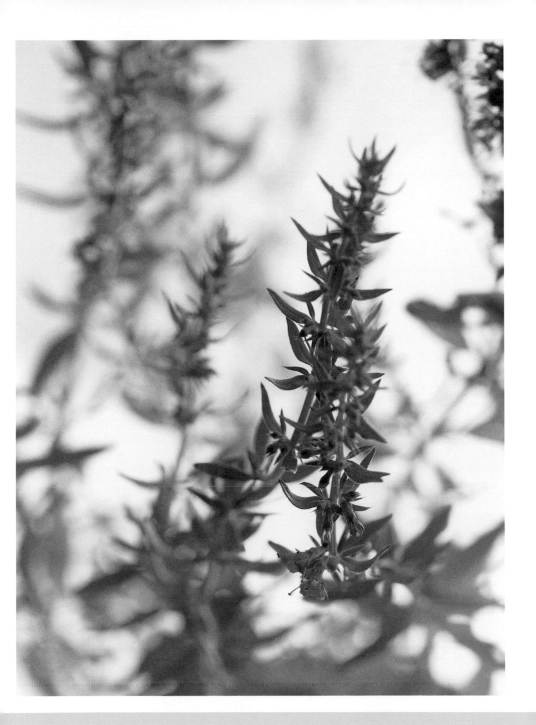

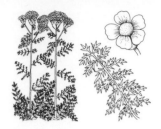
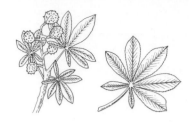

Achillea millefolium

Yarrow

Yarrow is a perennial herb native to Europe and Asia. It has been valued for stopping bleeding since the time of the ancient Greeks.

Family Asteraceae

Parts used Aerial Parts

Actions Diaphoretic, diuretic, astringent, digestive, bitter tonic, antimicrobial, decongestant, anti-inflammatory, antispasmodic, analgesic, antihistamine, emmenagogue, expectorant, haemostatic, alterative.

Digestion Stimulates appetite, aids digestion and absorption. • Relieves wind, spasm, IBS and indigestion. • Astringent tannins protect the gut from irritation and infection; helpful in diarrhoea and inflammatory problems.

Circulation Taken in hot tea it promotes sweating and reduces fevers. • Lowers blood pressure, improves circulation and relieves leg cramps and varicose veins.

Respiratory system Taken in hot tea with mint and elderflower it relieves colds and congestion. • Antihistamine effect is useful in treating allergies.

Immune system Volatile oils and luteolin have anti-inflammatory and antioxidant effects; relieve arthritis, allergies and autoimmune problems. • Clears toxins by aiding elimination via the skin and kidneys.

Urinary system Diuretic, relieves irritable bladder. Tightens muscles, helping incontinence.

Reproductive system Regulates menstrual cycle, relieves PMS and heavy bleeding.

Externally Tannins and silica speed healing of cuts, wounds, ulcers, burns, varicose veins, haemorrhoids and skin conditions.

CAUTION Avoid in pregnancy and if allergic to Asteraceae.

Drug interactions Avoid with anticoagulants.

Aesculus hippocastanum

Horse chestnut

This magnificent tree is native to western Asia and was brought to Europe in the mid-17th century. It is also found in North America. The extract of the seeds has long been valued in the treatment of vascular problems.

Family Hippocastanaceae

Parts used Seeds, bark

Actions Astringent, anti-inflammatory, febrifuge, anticoagulant, expectorant.

Digestion Bark is rich in astringent tannins, useful for treating diarrhoea.

Circulation Aescin strengthens blood vessel walls and enhances their elasticity, improving blood flow and venous return, and preventing pooling of blood causing piles and varicose veins. • Relieves pressure on the heart and high blood pressure. • Anticoagulant properties reduce blood clotting.

Immune system Saponin aescin has anti-inflammatory effects, helpful in easing joint pain. • Hot decoction reduces fevers; a traditional substitute for Peruvian Bark (Cinchona) for treating malaria and intermittent fevers.

Externally Contracts blood vessels and reduces fluid and swelling around areas of trauma, useful after surgery. • Creams or gels are excellent for treating varicose veins and ulcers, phlebitis and haemorrhoids, as well as cellulite. Can relieve the pain and swelling of arthritis, neuralgia, sunburn, bruises, sprains and other sports injuries.

CAUTION Avoid in pregnancy, lactation and children. All parts are toxic when raw; use pre-treated preparations and avoid large doses.

Drug interactions Avoid with anticoagulants and salicylates.

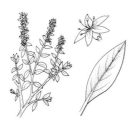
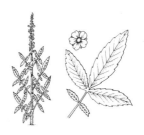

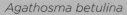

Agathosma betulina	*Agrimonia eupatoria*
# Buchu	# Agrimony

This woody evergreen shrub native to South Africa has highly aromatic leaves. It was used by the indigenous people to ward off insects and as an antiseptic for urinary tract infections, digestive problems, arthritis and gout.

Family Rutaceae

Parts used Leaves

Actions Antimicrobial, urinary antiseptic, diuretic, stimulating tonic, digestive, anti-inflammatory, depurative, astringent, carminative, diaphoretic, uterine stimulant.

Digestion Antimicrobial for treating infections such as gastroenteritis, diarrhoea and dysentery. • Relieves bloating, flatulence, stomach cramps and colic. • Helps regulate blood sugar.

Circulation May reduce blood pressure.

Immune system Anti-inflammatory and cleansing; helps the elimination of uric acid. Used in treating arthritis, gout, rheumatism and muscle aches. • Aids resistance to colds and flu; taken at onset of acute infections, chills and fevers.

Urinary system Effective diuretic, often included in formulae for PMS to relieve fluid retention. • Antibacterial and anti-inflammatory, used for treating urinary tract infections, cystitis, irritable bladder, stones, dysuria and haematuria. • Reduces acute and chronic inflammation and infection of the prostate.

Externally The oil is used as an insect repellent. • Used as a vaginal douche it allays yeast infections and leucorrhoea.

CAUTION Avoid in cases of acute inflammation of the liver and kidneys, and during pregnancy.

Drug interactions Avoid with warfarin and other anticoagulants.

This perennial plant native to Europe and northern Asia has spikes of yellow flowers and is named after the ancient Greek king Mithridates VI Eupator, who used it for treating liver problems and poisoning. It was valued on medieval battlefields for stopping bleeding.

Family Rosaceae

Parts used Aerial Parts

Actions Astringent, analgesic, anti-inflammatory, antispasmodic, antibacterial, digestive tonic, cholagogue, diuretic, emmenagogue, febrifuge, haemostatic.

Digestion Protects the gut lining from irritation and inflammation and counteracts infection. Used for peptic ulcers, gastritis, colitis and diarrhoea. • Bitters stimulate digestive juices and bile from the liver and gall bladder, enhancing digestion and absorption, improving bowel function. • Lowers blood sugar.

Respiratory system Antispamodic for asthma and coughs. • Antibacterial for infections and bronchitis.

Immune system Combats bacterial and viral infections. • Helps inhibit growth of tumours.

Urinary system Astringent diuretic for incontinence, bladder irritation, cystitis and kidney stones. • Aids elimination of uric acid, helpful for gout and arthritis.

Reproductive system Astringent for heavy periods.

Externally Gargle/mouthwash for sore throats, laryngitis and inflamed gums; eyebath for inflammatory eye problems; douche for vaginal infections • Stems bleeding, speeds healing of cuts, bruises, sprains and varicose veins; relieves aching muscles and skin problems.

Drug interactions Avoid with blood thinners such as warfarin; monitor with diabetic drugs and antihypertensives.

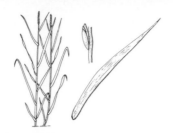

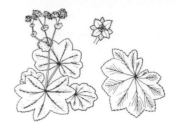

Agropyron repens
Couch grass

This perennial grass is native to Europe and North America. The rhizomes are a valuable remedy for urinary problems and can be ground into flour and roasted to make coffee.

Family Poaceae

Parts used Rhizomes

Actions Demulcent, emollient, diuretic, anti-inflammatory, antimicrobial, antifungal.

Digestion Soothes mucous membranes throughout the gut.

Circulation Reduces harmful cholesterol.

Respiratory system Soothing, antimicrobial and anti-inflammatory for irritating coughs, bronchitis and laryngitis. • Clears catarrhal congestion through its soothing effect on mucosa in the nose, throat and bronchi.

Musculoskeletal system Diuretic actions clear toxins, wastes and uric acid and helps relieve arthritis and gout. • Anti-inflammatory action is helpful in treating joint disease.

Immune system A traditional spring tonic, eliminates accumulated wastes via the kidneys. • Clears heat and reduces fevers.

Urinary system Abundant mucilage soothes the urinary tract. • Mannitol acts as an osmotic diuretic, saponins and vanillin are also diuretic, aiding the excretion of wastes including excess sodium and uric acid. • Used for treating infections and inflammatory conditions such as cystitis, irritable bladder, dysuria, haematuria, urethritis, prostatitis (acute and chronic) and benign enlargement of prostate. • Silicic acid is healing and strengthening to the urinary tract and sphincters, used for urinary incontinence.

Externally Gargle used for sore throats, laryngitis, tonsillitis; soothing wash for inflammation, eczema, cuts and grazes.

Alchemilla vulgaris
Lady's mantle

Lady's mantle is a distinctive perennial native to Europe and northern Asia.

Family Rosaceae

Parts used Root, leaves, flowers

Actions Astringent, haemostatic, anti-inflammatory, diuretic, emmenagogue, febrifuge.

Digestion Astringent for diarrhoea and inflammatory problems such as gastritis, colitis and gastroenteritis.

Urinary system Cools heat and inflammation and relieves cystitis.

Reproductive system Astringent and anti-inflammatory for heavy, painful and irregular periods, prolonged bleeding due to fibroids or during menopause. • Used to promote fertility. • Toning for weak pelvic floor muscles, helps prevent miscarriage and good for treating prolapse. • Used to aid contractions during childbirth, speed recovery and regulate hormones and strengthen muscles after miscarriage and childbirth. Taken a few days prior to birth helps prevent post-partum bleeding. • Cooling and balancing remedy during menopause. • For fibroids, genito-urinary infections, endometriosis and pelvic inflammatory disease.

Externally Astringent fresh root/leaves stop bleeding and promote healing. • Gargle/mouthwash used for mouth ulcers and sores, sore throats and laryngitis. • Lotion used for skin problems such as inflamed cuts and abrasions, pimples or rashes; eyewash for conjunctivitis. • Douche used for vaginal irritation and infections such as candida and after-antibiotic treatment for infection such as trichomonas, when the vaginal flora has been disturbed.

CAUTION Avoid during pregnancy, except in the last few weeks.

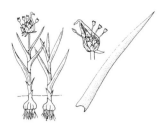
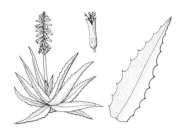

Allium sativum
Garlic

This excellent antimicrobial herb has been prescribed since the 1st century CE by Ayurvedic doctors for infections. Its antibiotic activity was noted by Louis Pasteur.

Family Alliaceae

Parts used Bulb

Actions Carminative, expectorant, alterative, immunostimulant, antimicrobial, anthelmintic, hypocholesterolaemic, hypotensive, antitumour, rejuvenative, circulatory stimulant, digestive.

Digestion Stimulates digestion and absorption. • May benefit type 2 diabetes.

Circulation Increases circulation and reduces blood pressure. Used for cramps and disorders such as Raynaud's disease. • Lowers harmful cholesterol and triglyceride levels. • Reduces tendency to clotting and reduces the risk of heart attacks and strokes.

Respiratory system Antimicrobial for chest infections, colds and flu. • Expectorant and decongestant; clears catarrh, sinusitis, coughs, asthma, hay fever and rhinitis.

Immune system Antibacterial, antifungal and antiviral, particularly for the respiratory, digestive and urinary systems. Active against viruses, including influenza B and herpes simplex type 1 and 2. • Powerful antioxidant; slows ageing process. • Sulphur compounds have antitumour activities and protect against pollution and nicotine.

Externally Oil/ointment used for cuts, wounds, arthritis, sprains, unbroken chilblains, athlete's foot, stings and warts. • Eardrops used for middle ear infection.

CAUTION Avoid large doses during pregnancy. May cause gastrointestinal upset. Applied to skin can cause dermatitis.

Drug interactions Avoid large doses with warfarin and antihypertensives.

Aloe barbadensis
Aloe vera

Indigenous to East and South Africa, this perennial succulent grows happily in most tropical places.

Family Aloaceae

Parts used Gel of inner leaves

Actions Demulcent, immunostimulant, anti-inflammatory, alterative, analgesic, antihistamine, antibacterial, antiviral, antiseptic, anthelmintic, digestive, rejuvenative, antioxidant, hypoglycaemic, diuretic.

Digestion Mild laxative; clears toxins and heat from the bowel. • Combats pathogenic micro-organisms. • Enhances the secretion of digestive enzymes and balances stomach acid. • Regulates sugar and fat metabolism. • Soothes and protects the gut lining; used for colitis, peptic ulcers, IBS and inflammatory bowel disease.

Musculoskeletal system Anti-inflammatory and detoxifying for arthritis.

Immune system Acemannan enhances immunity, is antiviral and stimulates activity of B- and T-lymphocytes, helping to destroy malignant cells. • Sterols have an anti-inflammatory action. • Antiviral for herpes simplex and zoster (shingles). • Used as a probiotic to treat candida.

Reproductive system Increases blood to the uterus. • Reduces hot flushes during menopause. • Used to treat PMS.

Externally Soothes and heals burns, sunburn, wounds, haemorrhoids and skin conditions such as acne, eczema and psoriasis. • Antibacterial, antifungal and antiviral. • Rejuvenates skin and reduces wrinkles. • Excellent for sensitive and allergic skin conditions.

CAUTION Drug interactions Possible interaction with cardiac glycosides and steroids.

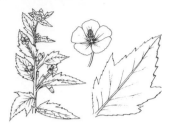
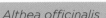
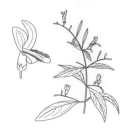

Althea officinalis
Marshmallow

This stately perennial grows in marshes by the sea in Europe and western Asia. Marshmallow cools irritation and inflammation – ideal for treating sore or inflamed mucous membranes.

Family Malvaceae

Parts used Root, leaf, flower

Actions Emollient, demulcent, anti-inflammatory, analgesic, antiseptic, antitussive, expectorant, diuretic, immune enhancer.

Digestion Anti-inflammatory for ulcerative colitis, gastritis and peptic ulcers. • Mucilage soothes heartburn, IBS and constipation from dryness. • Reduces peristalsis and relieves diarrhoea; larger doses have a mild laxative effect.

Respiratory system Mild expectorant and immune enhancer. Soothes harsh, dry coughs, sore throats, laryngitis, bronchitis and croup; clears catarrh and alleviates inflammation.

Immune system Stimulates production of white blood cells.

Urinary system Soothing diuretic, relieving cystitis, urethritis and irritable bladder. Eases passing of gravel and stones.

Reproductive system Traditionally added to prescriptions to ease childbirth. • Stimulates flow of breast milk.

Externally Leaves are applied to irritation and inflammation from insect bites and wasp and bee stings. • Used with lavender and flax oil for treating scalds and burns and sunburn. • Soothes and heals inflamed skin in sore nipples, acne and eczema. • Warm poultice used to draw out splinters and for mastitis, boils and abscesses. • Mouthwash/gargle used to treat sore throats and inflamed gums.

Andrographis paniculata
Andrographis

Native to India and cultivated in China, this annual has a very bitter taste and is highly valued in Ayurvedic medicine for enhancing immunity and combating acute infection.

Family Acanthaceae

Parts used Aerial parts

Actions Immunostimulant, antimicrobial, choleretic, hepatoprotective, febrifuge, anodyne, antiparasitic, anthelmintic.

Digestion Antiviral, antiprotazoal, antifungal, antiparasitic and anthelmintic. Helps re-establish normal gut flora and combat acute infections, bacillary dysentery, enteritis, worms, parasites and candida. • Antibacterial against Staphylococcus aureus, Pseudomonas aeruginosa, Proteus vulgaris, Shigella dysenteriae and E. coli. • Bitter and cooling, it enhances digestion, stimulates bile flow from the liver and protects the liver from damage by toxins, alcohol and infections such as hepatitis. • Anti-inflammatory for indigestion, heartburn, acidity, flatulence, gastritis, colitis and peptic ulcers.

Respiratory system For throat and ear infections, coughs, colds, flu, acute bronchitis and chest infections with fever. • Reduces phlegm; helpful in asthma.

Immune system Immune enhancing; excellent for the prevention and treatment of infections such as colds, flu, coughs, sinusitis, mouth ulcers, shingles, otitis media, sore throats, laryngitis, tonsilitis and septic conditions of the blood. • Useful for leptospirosis, high fevers and malaria. • Protects the liver and inhibits platelet aggregation.

Urinary system For heat and infection of the urinary tract from dysuria, haematuria and proteinuria.

Externally Used as a wash/cream for inflamed and infected skin problems such as acne, eczema, spots and boils.

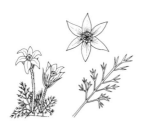

Anemone pulsatilla
Pasque flower

Despite its delicate appearance, the Pasque flower it is remarkably resilient, flowering in early spring but often in very wintery weather.

Family Ranunculaceae

Parts used Dried aerial parts

Actions Analgesic, sedative, antispasmodic, decongestant, febrifuge.

Circulation Improves venous circulation; for varicose veins and nosebleeds.

Mental and emotional Excellent relaxant and nerve tonic. Promotes relaxation and sleep and facilitates recovery when run-down by conserving energy.
• Used for nervous exhaustion, depression, insomnia, nightmares, irritability, weepiness, clinginess and fear of being alone. • Used for PMS, overexcitement, weepiness, depression after childbirth and during menopause.

Respiratory system Astringent and antibacterial; used for colds, acute and chronic catarrh and coughs.

Musculoskeletal system Relieves spasm and excellent for reducing pain; used for colic, period pain, headaches, asthma and neuralgia.

Immune system In hot infusion relieves fevers, brings out rash in eruptive infections such as measles and speeds recovery.

Reproductive system Specific for pain and inflammation in men and women. • Used for afterpains and post-natal depression. • Tonic and relaxant properties help regulate contractions. • Used for PMS and menopausal depression.

Eyes and ears Used for painful inflammatory eye conditions including scleritis, iritis, glaucoma and cataracts. • Used for otitis media and earache.

CAUTION Avoid during pregnancy.

Anethum graveolens
Dill

This highly aromatic annual is originally from the Mediterranean. Its name is said to come from the Saxon word dilla, meaning 'to lull', due to its ability to relax children into a restful sleep.

Family Apiaceae

Parts used Leaf, seed

Actions Carminative, alterative, expectorant, diuretic, antispasmodic, vermifuge, analgesic, relaxant, digestive, sedative, anti-inflammatory, antioxidant, antimicrobial.

Digestion Stimulates appetite and digestion.
• Releases tension and spasm; used for colic, wind, indigestion, nausea, constipation and diarrhoea.

Mental and emotional Helps alleviate tiredness from disturbed nights and enhances concentration and memory. • Relaxant for insomnia and stress-related digestive disorders such as wind, colic and constipation.

Respiratory system Antispasmodic and expectorant for harsh, dry coughs and asthma.

Musculoskeletal system Volatile oil in the leaves and seeds relaxes smooth muscle. Good for relieving tension and pain.

Immune system Research has confirmed its antibacterial and anticandida properties. • May inhibit cancer formation.

Urinary system It has diuretic effects.

Reproductive system Used for painful periods.
• In the East it is given to women prior to childbirth to ease childbirth. • Increases milk in breast-feeding women.

Externally Analgesic and anti-inflammatory properties relieve pain and swelling. • Essential oil in massage oils and liniments used to treat abdominal pain, colic, arthritis and earache.

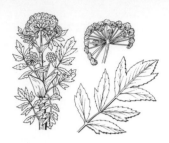

Angelica archangelica
Angelica

This statuesque biennial, native to parts of Europe, was historically valued for its protection against poisoning, contagion and witches.

Family Apiaceae

Parts used Dried root, leaf, stem, seed

Actions Antibacterial, antifungal, alterative, anti-inflammatory, carminative, diaphoretic, digestive, diuretic, tonic, circulatory stimulant, antispasmodic, expectorant, emmenagogue.

Digestion Stimulates digestion; used for weak digestion, nausea, indigestion, wind and colic.
• Inhaling the crushed leaves relieves travel sickness.
• Improves appetite, metabolism and absorption.
• Taken regularly it is traditionally thought to reduce the desire for alcohol.

Circulation Warming circulatory tonic; stimulates blood flow to the periphery; excellent for problems with poor circulation such as Raynaud's disease and Buerger's disease. • Calcium-channel blocker in the heart; useful for high blood pressure and angina.
• Used to treat anaemia.

Mental and emotional Strengthening nerve tonic; aids inspiration. • Mood elevating in depression.

Respiratory system Warming expectorant and decongestant for coughs, acute bronchitis, asthma, sore throats, colds and catarrh. • Hot tea helps to relieve fevers.

Immune system Antimicrobial and cleansing; aids detoxification and enhances immunity. • Anti-inflammatory for arthritis and gout.

Reproductive system Regulates menstrual cycle and relieves period pain and PMS.

Externally Used in massage oils or baths to relieve muscle tension and joint stiffness and pain.

CAUTION Avoid fresh root during pregnancy. May cause photosensitivity.

Angelica polymorph var. sinensis
Chinese angelica/Dong guai

This perennial herb is found in the mountain forests of China, Japan and Korea. It is an important blood and liver tonic in Traditional Chinese Medicine.

Family Apiaceae

Parts used Root

Actions Emmenagogue, antiviral, antibacterial, antifungal, antispasmodic, circulatory stimulant, digestive, alterative, analgesic, anti-inflammatory, decongestant, diuretic, immunostimulant, tonic.

Digestion Warming digestive stimulant; increases appetite and digestion. Used for constipation.

Circulation Decreases blood pressure, regulates the heart, inhibits platelet aggregation, reduces atherosclerosis, enhances circulation and dilates coronary arteries. • Used for angina, arrhythmias, palpitations, atrial fibrillation, Buerger's disease, Raynaud's syndrome and cramps.

Mental and emotional Mild analgesic for headaches, neuralgia and shingles pain. • Strengthening tonic for exhaustion. • Relaxant for insomnia.

Respiratory system Clears catarrh and asthma.

Immune system Stimulates formation of white blood cells, lymphocytes and phagocytes. • For herpes infections and malaria. • Protects the liver. • Inhibits immunoglobulin E antibodies in allergies.

Urinary system Diuretic; relieves fluid retention. Useful for dispelling premenstrual fluid accumulation.

Reproductive system Balances hormones. • Renowned women's tonic for menstrual irregularities, dysmenorrhoea, PMS and heavy periods. • Enhances fertility. • Aids contractions during childbirth. • Used for menopausal symptoms such as night sweats, hot flushes, depression and mood swings.

CAUTION Avoid during pregnancy.

Drug interactions Avoid with anticoagulants.

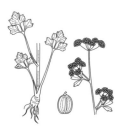
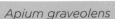
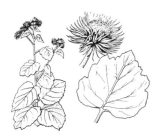

Apium graveolens
Wild celery

This aromatic biennial, native to the Mediterranean, is believed to be the original celery. It has been popular since Roman times for relieving aches and pains.

Family Apiaceae

Parts used Seeds

Actions Diuretic, urinary antiseptic, antioxidant, hypotensive, depurative, antibacterial, antifungal, sedative, antispasmodic, uterotonic, antineoplastic, anti-inflammatory, immunostimulant, analgesic.

Digestion Antispasmodic and digestive; enhances appetite, digestion and absorption and relieves spasm, colic, indigestion, hiccups, heartburn and nausea.

Circulation Reduces circulating dopamine, norepinephrine and epinephrine, helping to reduce blood pressure. • Antiplatelet effects; reduces the formation of clots and helps prevent heart attacks.

Mental and emotional Calming and uplifting; used for stress-related headaches, mental and physical tiredness, insomnia, depression, agitation and panic. • Releases muscle tension and spasm.

Musculoskeletal system Excellent anti-inflammatory for arthritis, rheumatism and gout. • A diuretic that dissolves and excretes uric acid. • Relieves muscle pain, tension and spasm. • Reduces neuralgia and sciatica.

Immune system Enhances immunity; antimicrobial effects help ward off colds, flu, asthma and bronchitis.

Urinary system Apiol is a urinary antiseptic. • Relieves fluid retention and cystitis; helps to eliminate toxins. • Prevents the formation of stones and gravel.

Reproductive system Enhances milk supply in lactating mothers. • Uterine stimulant; brings on periods and stimulates contractions in childbirth.

CAUTION Avoid in pregnancy and with kidney inflammation.

Arctium lappa
Burdock

A biennial native to temperate Europe and northern Asia, respected for its detoxifying and antiseptic properties.

Family Asteraceae

Parts used Root, seed, leaf

Actions Alterative, diaphoretic, demulcent, diuretic, astringent, bitter tonic, digestive, mild laxative, antimicrobial, hypoglycaemic, antitumour, probiotic.

Digestion Enhances digestion and liver function, mild laxative and depurative. Relieves wind, distension and indigestion. • Hypoglycaemic action; helpful for diabetes. • Mucilaginous fibres absorb toxins from the gut and enhance their elimination from the bowel. • Used for bacterial and fungal infections; fructooligosaccharides in the root have a probiotic effect.

Respiratory system Enhances immunity to infections. • Used for sore throats, swollen glands and tonsils.

Immune system Antibacterial, antifungal and antitumour. • In hot decoction it reduces fevers, clears toxins via the skin, brings out eruptions and speeds recovery from measles and chickenpox. • Cleansing for chronic inflammatory conditions such as gout, arthritis and rheumatism and skin problems.

Urinary system Aids elimination of toxins via urine. • Used for cystitis, water retention, stones and gravel.

Reproductive system Root stimulates the uterus, aids liver function and the breakdown of hormones and helps regulate periods. • Traditionally used for prolapse. • Imparts strength before and after childbirth.

Skin Used for chronic skin disease such as acne; improves action of the sebaceous glands.

CAUTION Avoid in pregnancy.

Drug interactions Avoid with antidiabetic drugs as it may have hypoglycaemic effects.

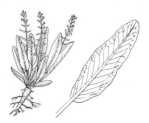
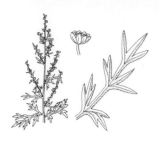

Armoracia rusticana
Horseradish

Native to southeastern Europe and western Asia, this perennial herb has a white tapered root that when cut or grated releases its strong aroma and powerfully acrid properties.

Family Brassicaceae

Parts used Fresh root

Actions Circulatory stimulant, decongestant, digestive, antimicrobial, expectorant, alterative, anthelmintic, diuretic, anti-inflammatory.

Digestion Enhances appetite, digestion and absorption. • Traditionally used as horseradish sauce to accompany roast beef because it stimulates the flow of gastric juices that break down heavy, indigestible foods and prevents indigestion.

Circulation Horseradish is a powerful stimulant, improving circulation and useful in disorders such as Raynaud's disease and Buerger's disease.

Respiratory system Stimulates mucous membranes; acts as a decongestant and expectorant, clearing catarrh and blocked sinuses. • Antimicrobial properties help combat infection. • Relieves coughs, colds, fevers, flu, sinusitis and hay fever.

Musculoskeletal system Hastens the elimination of toxins; recommended for gout and arthritis.

Immune system Antibiotic properties; excellent for respiratory and urinary infections.

Urinary system Asparagin is diuretic; relieves fliud retention and clears toxins via the kidneys.

Other Stimulating, heating energy tonic, excellent in winter for warding off the cold.

CAUTION May irritate the eyes and skin when grating/cutting the fresh root. Avoid in pregnancy and with thyroid problems and symptoms characterized by heat such as gastritis and peptic ulcers.

Artemisia absinthium
Wormwood

This aromatic perennial is native to Europe, western Asia and North Africa. Intensely bitter and aromatic, it is strengthening and reviving, stimulating the stomach, gall bladder and liver.

Family Asteraceae

Parts used Aerial parts

Actions Bitter tonic, digestive, anthelmintic, alterative, antiseptic, anti-inflammatory, anodyne, immunostimulant, antifungal, cholagogue, antiemetic, diuretic, emmenagogue, insecticide.

Digestion Stimulates the flow of hydrochloric acid and enhances appetite, digestion, absorption and liver function. • Used for heartburn, acidity, liver problems, halitosis, gastritis, indigestion, anorexia, flatulence, nausea, vomiting, diarrhoea and gastroenteritis. • Taken on an empty stomach for treating pin worms. • Antimicrobial for food poisoning.

Mental and emotional Stimulates the brain. • Traditionally used for neuralgia, depression and nervous exhaustion.

Musculoskeletal system Anti-inflammatory for gout and arthritis.

Immune system Volatile oils are strongly antibacterial. • Enhances immunity and clears toxins; good when run-down or recovering from illness. • Taken hot for fevers, colds and flu and to clear catarrh.

Reproductive system Stimulates uterine muscles, brings on periods and aids contractions during childbirth. • Regulates the menstrual cycle, relieves painful periods and promotes fertility.

Externally A wash used for fleas and lice; lotion for skin problems such as nappy rash, athlete's foot, scabies and boils, and hair loss, bruises, sprains and arthritic pain.

CAUTION Avoid during pregnancy and breastfeeding. Low doses are recommended, for example, 0.25–1 ml of tincture 3 x daily or 1–2 g dried herb 3 x daily.

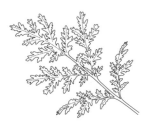

Artemisia annua
Sweet Annie

Native to Asia and eastern Europe, this annual feathery herb is found throughout temperate and subtropical areas. Artemisinin, a key active component, is popular as an effective remedy for malaria.

Family Asteraceae

Parts used Leaf

Actions Bitter, carminative, digestive, antiparasitic, febrifuge, antimalarial, antiseptic, antibacterial, anti-inflammatory, digestive.

Digestion Enhances appetite and digestion; relieves wind and indigestion. • Recommended for infections including salmonella, dysentery and diarrhoea.

Respiratory system Infusion of the leaves is used to treat fevers, chills, colds and other infections.

Immune system Clears heat; reduces fevers from infections and sunstroke. • Antimicrobial for TB and other infections. • Enhances immunity, reduces inflammation and may be helpful in autoimmune disease. Studies using 50 g herb or 0.3 g artemisinin daily have shown it to improve symptoms in systemic lupus erythematosus. • Qinghaoic acid is antibacterial against, for example, Staphylococcus aureus, E. coli and Salmonella typhosa. • Artemisinin releases free radicals once inside red blood cells that kill malaria parasites. • Artemisinin is effective against drug-resistant Plasmodium spp. Research has shown its efficacy in treating malaria, but other constituents may contribute. • May have anticancer properties, particularly in relation to breast and prostate cancer and leukaemia.

Externally Poultice of the leaves is applied to nosebleeds, abscesses and boils. • In China the leaves are burned as a fumigant insecticide to kill mosquitoes.

CAUTION Avoid in pregnancy. May cause contact dermatitis.

Asclepias tuberosa
Pleurisy root

Native to North America, Pleurisy root was used by Native American tribes as a remedy for chest infections and externally to treat wounds.

Family Asclepiadaceae

Parts used Root

Actions Diaphoretic, vasorelaxant, febrifuge, antispasmodic, amphoteric, expectorant, anti-inflammatory, antiviral, antimicrobial, expectorant, carminative, cathartic, diuretic.

Digestion Antispasmodic and soothing; relieves flatulence, colic and irritation of the gut lining that causes indigestion and diarrhoea.

Circulation Traditionally used for pericarditis and to slow down a rapid pulse. • Relaxes arteries, brings blood to the periphery and promotes sweating; relieves pressure in the heart and arteries.

Mental and emotional Calms the nerves and relaxes tense muscles.

Respiratory system Promotes sweating in fevers and flu. • Expectorant for coughs; helps clear catarrh. • Its antispasmodic properties are helpful in asthma and emphysema. • Relieves pain, infection and inflammation in bronchitis, laryngitis, croup, pneumonia, hoarsness and chest infections including pneumonia. • Reabsorbs pleural effusion from the pleura; specific for pleurisy, pleuritic pain and dry, painful coughs.

Skin Brings out rash in eruptive diseases including measles and chickenpox.

CAUTION Large doses may cause diarrhoea and vomiting. Avoid in pregnancy and breastfeeding.

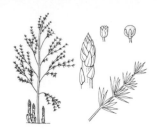
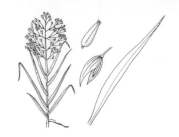

Asparagus racemosus
Shatavari/Wild asparagus

This perennial is similar in appearance to cultivated asparagus.

Family Asparagaceae

Parts used Leaf, root

Actions Tonic, rejuvenative, adaptogen, antispasmodic, anti-inflammatory, demulcent, refrigerant, diuretic, aphrodisiac, tonic, expectorant, antibacterial, alterative, antitumour, antacid.

Digestion Cooling and demulcent for dry, inflamed mucous membranes, dyspepsia, gastritis, peptic ulcers and inflammatory bowel problems such as Crohn's disease and IBS. • Relieves diarrhoea and dysentery.

Mental and emotional Valued in India for promoting memory and mental clarity. • For ADHD in children combined with brain tonics such as Centella asiatica (Gotu kola). • Reduces anxiety and stress. • Increases energy and strength.

Respiratory system Soothes sore throats, dry coughs and irritated conditions.

Immune system Enhances immunity, growth and development in babies and children.• Enhances the ability to fight infections and the production of immune-regulating messenger molecules • Protects blood-producing cells in the bone marrow, aiding recovery after exposure to toxic chemicals. • Antibacterial activity including E. Coli, Shigella spp., Salmonella spp. and Pseudomonas; antiviral against herpes. • Anti-inflammatory for gout and arthritis.

Urinary system Soothing and cooling for cystitis. • Dissolves stones and gravel. • Reduces fluid retention.

Reproductive system Enhances fertility; used for low libido and sperm count. • Regulates hormonal imbalances; useful during menopause. • Increases milk production.

Externally Used for swollen joints and muscle tension; ingredient of mahanarayan oil for joint and muscle pain. • Reduces development of scar tissue after surgery.

Avena sativa
Wild oats

An annual grass native to Europe, Asia and North Africa, oats are highly nutritious, full of protein, calcium, magnesium, silica, iron and vitamins, which are strengthening to bones and teeth and vital to a healthy nervous system.

Family Poaceae

Parts used Whole plant, seed

Actions Sedative, antidepressant, diuretic, antispasmodic, demulcent, laxative, nutritive, rejuvenative, antilipidemic, hypocholesterolaemic, antidiabetic.

Digestion For constipation; help prevent bowel cancer by removing toxins from the bowel. • Since they lower blood sugar, they are useful for diabetics.

Circulation Lower blood cholesterol and help combat cardiovascular problems; oat bran fibre binds to cholesterol and bile components to be excreted via the bowels.

Mental and emotional Good tonic for the nervous system, supporting the body during times of stress, relieving depression, anxiety, tension and nervous exhaustion. • Worth taking when withdrawing from tranquillizers and antidepressants. Oat green tea is used for drug, alcohol and nicotine addiction. • May decrease the hypertensive effects of nicotine.

Reproductive system Regulate hormones in the body, notably oestrogen.

Externally Oatmeal makes a good facial scrub and soothing remedy for irritated and inflamed skin conditions.

Drug interactions May decrease the effects of morphine.

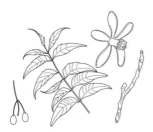
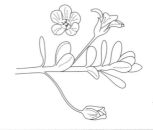

Azadirachta indica
Neem

This evergreen tree native to Southeast Asia is primarily used for combating infections and inflammation.

Family Meliaceae

Parts used Flower, seed, leaf, bark

Actions Febrifuge, antiseptic, anthelmintic, anti-inflammatory, expectorant, hypoglycaemic, antimicrobial, antifertility, alterative, antibacterial, antifungal, antiviral, astringent, bitter, emmenagogue.

Digestion Stimulates appetite, digestion and enhances liver function. • Hepatoprotective activity protects the liver from injury from toxins, drugs, chemotherapy and viruses. • Regulates blood sugar in diabetes.

Circulation Reduces serum cholesterol levels and blood pressure and regulates the heart.

Mental and emotional Reduces anxiety, stress, anger, irritability, intolerance and depression. • Relieves pain.

Respiratory system Decongestant, expectorant and antimicrobial; clears infection and phlegm.

Immune system Leaves and bark are antibacterial, antifungal and antiparasitic. • Used in the prevention and treatment of malaria. • Used for inflammatory arthritis.

Reproductive system Stimulates uterine muscle; used for delayed and painful childbirth and as a tonic after birth.

Skin For skin disorders, eczema, acne, boils, psoriasis, abscesses and haemorrhoids.

Externally For infections such as chickenpox, head lice and athlete's foot. Widely used in non-toxic insecticides. • In liniments for joint pain and muscle aches.

CAUTION Avoid in pregnancy and lactation. May reduce fertility and cause hypersensitivity reactions.

Drug interactions Use with care in patients on insulin.

Bacopa monnieri
Brahmi

Native to India and other tropical regions, Brahmi derives its name from Brahman, meaning 'pure consciousness', because of its ability to aid meditation.

Family Scrophulariaceae

Parts used Dried whole plant, mainly leaf and stalk

Actions Adaptogen, antidepressant, anxiolytic, diuretic, sedative, rejuvenative, antispasmodic, carminative, bronchial dilator, anticonvulsant, immunostimulant, anti-inflammatory, antiseptic, antifungal, antioxidant, antirheumatic, diuretic.

Digestion Suppresses appetite; best combined with warming digestive herbs such as Ginger and Cardamom. • Astringent for stress-related diarrhoea and IBS.

Mental and emotional Used in India and China to enhance brain function and learning ability, improve memory and concentration and calm anxiety and mental turbulence. • Enhances neurotransmitter/synapse function and increases serotonin production and brain cell activity. Helpful for ADD, ADHD, learning and behavioural problems, hyperactivity, Alzheimer's disease, epilepsy, mental illness, restlessness, insomnia and anxiety. • Increases resilience to stress, combats nervous exhaustion and relieves depression. • Hersaponin, one of four saponins, has sedative properties.

Respiratory system For coughs and colds, bronchitis, asthma and hoarseness. • Poultice of the boiled plant can be applied to the chest for bronchitis and chronic cough.

Urinary system Cooling diuretic; used for cystitis and irritable bladder. • Nourishing kidney tonic.

Other • Relieves joint pain. • Helps chelate heavy metals from the body.

Externally Oil/fresh leaf juice is used for joint pain. • Applied to the head to clear the mind and relieve headaches.

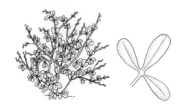
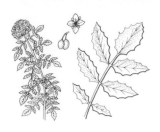

Baptisia tinctoria
Wild indigo

This North American perennial plant has bright yellow flowers. It was popular among American physicians in the early 1900s as an 'epidemic remedy' to combat infections.

Family Fabaceae

Parts used Root, leaf

Actions Lymphatic, antipyretic, immune enhancing, alterative, antibiotic, anti-inflammatory, antiseptic, antiviral, astringent, emmenagogue, laxative, stimulant.

Digestion Laxative; clears toxins and infection from the bowel. • Used for acute infections, gastroenteritis and bacterial dysentery. • Traditionally used for typhoid.

Respiratory system Antibacterial and antiviral; helps ward off and treat infections of the ear, nose, throat and chest. • Useful for treating chronic bronchitis.

Immune system • Potent antimicrobial for acute and chronic infections. Polysaccharides stimulate phagocytosis, enhancing immunity. • Used at the onset of colds, flu, fevers, infections of the respiratory and digestive system, herpes, glandular fever, tonsillitis and laryngitis. • Good remedy for chronic fatigue syndrome. • Indicated in immunization reactions. • May have antimalarial and anticancer activity.

Urinary system Antimicrobial for chronic cystitis.

Skin Cleansing and antimicrobial for infected skin problems including boils, abscesses, Staphylococcus aureus infections, warts and impetigo.

Externally Poultice used for spots, boils, acne, eczema, Staphylococcus aureus infections, warts, cuts and wounds. • Mouthwash/gargle used for inflammation or infection of gums, mouth ulcers and sore throat. • Used as a douche for cervicitis, vaginal discharge, candida and vaginitis.

Berberis aquifolium
Oregon grape root

Native to western North America, this root was traditionally used by Native Americans as a detoxifier for infections and skin problems.

Family Berberidaceae

Parts used Dried root, rhizome

Actions Alterative, bitter tonic, cholagogue, digestive, laxative, astringent, antiseptic, antitumour, diuretic, thyroid stimulant, antioxidant.

Digestion Used for treating hepatitis and gallstones. • Bitters stimulate the flow of saliva, digestive enzymes and bile. • Clears toxins and relieves constipation. • Clears infections, diarrhoea, dysentery, Shigella spp., Staphylococcus aureus, Salmomella spp. and dysbiosis. • Used for headaches and malaise associated with toxicity. • Increases stamina.

Circulation Reduces venous congestion; improves varicose veins and haemorrhoids. • Dilates blood vessels and reduces blood pressure. • For anaemia; releases stored iron from the liver.

Mental and emotional Cooling remedy for fiery people who are critical, self-critical and dissatisfied.

Musculoskeletal system Anti-inflammatory and depurative for gout, rheumatism and arthritis.

Immune system Berberine enhances immunity against a wide range of microbes and inhibits tumour development.

Urinary system Diuretic; aids cleansing by enhancing the elimination of toxins.

Reproductive system Reduces blood congestion that causes heavy periods and menstrual pain.

Skin Clears toxins, heat and inflammation, acne, boils, herpes, eczema and psoriasis.

Externally Compress or poultice used for boils and irritation of the skin. • Gargle used for sore throats.

CAUTION Avoid in hyperthyroidism and during pregnancy. Fresh roots/rhizomes are purgative.

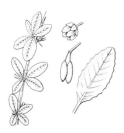
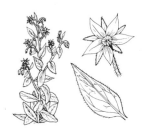

Berberis vulgaris
Barberry

Native to temperate climates, this shrub is found growing wild in Europe and North America. One of the best cleansing herbs, the root was traditionally used by Native Americans and in European folk medicine for infections, liver and stomach ailments and as a general tonic during convalescence.

Family Berberidaceae

Parts used Root, stem/bark

Actions Antimicrobial, cholagogue, choleretic, antiemetic, bitter tonic, antiparasitic, probiotic.

Digestion Maintains normal gut flora and combats infection in the gut including E. coli and amoebic dysentery, Giardia, Blastocystis hominis and Dientamoeba fragilis. Inhibits endotoxins. • Bitters stimulate bile flow from the liver and help detoxify the body. • Indicated for viral liver infections and gall bladder problems.

Circulation Regulates the heart and decreases ventricular arrhythmias and palpitations. • Increases platelets in thrombocytopenia.

Musculoskeletal system Anti-inflammatory and detoxyifing remedy for arthritis, rheumatism and gout.

Immune system Antioxidant; reduces oxygen free radicals and helps protect against cancer. • Potent antimicrobial active against bacteria, fungi, viruses, worms and chlamydia. • Berberine is active against Staphylococcus epidermidis, E. coli and Neisseria meningitides. • Indicated in acute bowel infection, diarrhoea, dysentery and cholera. • Decreases inflammation and has an antihistamine action, useful in infected skin conditions such as boils and abscesses and allergies, including hay fever, atopic eczema and asthma, and migraine.

Externally Cream used for psoriasis. • Used in a saline solution as eye drops.

Borago officinalis
Borage

Native to Europe, Asia and North Africa, borage is a perennial with bright blue flowers and leaves that smell like cucumber. It is good for cooling inflammation and clearing toxins.

Family Boraginaceae

Parts used Leaf, flower, seed oil

Actions Leaf and flower: expectorant, diuretic, adrenal tonic, alterative, decongestant, demulcent, anti-inflammatory, antihypertensive, diaphoretic; seed oil: antiarthritic, anti-inflammatory, antihypertensive, hormone regulator.

Circulation GLA in seed oil converts in the body to prostaglandin E1 (PGE1), which dilates blood vessels, reduces blood pressure and blood clots and lowers harmful cholesterol.

Mental and emotional Relieves tension and anxiety, increases resilience to stress, supports adrenals, lifts spirits and improves mental energy.

Respiratory system Decongestant and soothing expectorant for catarrh, coughs, bronchitis, pneumonia and pleurisy. • GLA reduces inflammation of the lungs and improves oxygenation; helpful in asthma, bronchitis and chronic airways obstruction.

Immune system Increases sweat and urine production; clears heat and toxins. • GLA has anti-inflammatory properties; relieves eczema and other skin inflammation. • GLA is useful for diabetes, scleroderma, Sjögren's syndrome and to slow ageing • GLA is helpful in prostate cancer, allergies and inflammatory arthritis.

Urinary system Cools and soothes irritation and inflammation; relieves cystitis, urinary tract infections and fluid retention.

Reproductive system Increases milk flow in nursing mothers. • GLA is useful for PMS, menstrual problems and menopause.

Externally Compress used for inflamed eyes and skin and bruises; gargle for sore throats.

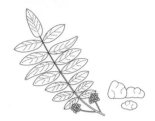
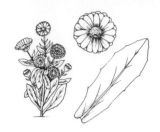

Boswellia serrata
Frankincense

Native to North Africa and the Middle East, the scored bark of frankincense secretes a juice that hardens into a brown resin used for medicine and incense.

Family Burseraceae

Parts used Gum resin from bark

Actions Anti-inflammatory, antiarthritic, antitumour, aphrodisiac, analgesic, hypocholesterolaemic, emmenagogue, antispasmodic.

Digestion Anti-inflamatory, used for colitis, Crohn's disease and ulcerative colitis.

Circulation Improves blood flow to the joints, prevents breakdown of tissues. • Reduces harmful cholesterol, clears ama from the blood. • Traditionally used for relieving pain and arthritis, and for psoriasis. • Reduces inflammation and inhibits the formation of tumours.

Mental and emotional Opens the mind; valued for its specific effect on the spiritual centre connected with the pituitary and hypothalamus gland.

Respiratory system Clears catarrh, coughs, bronchitis and asthma.

Musculoskeletal system Speeds the healing of broken bones. • Inhibits the breakdown of connective tissue, increases blood supply to the joints and strengthens blood vessels.

Reproductive system Used for uterine congestion, fibroids, cysts and painful periods with clots. • Brings blood to the penis and improves erectile function. • Good alternative to non-steroidal anti-inflammatory drugs for rheumatoid arthritis, osteoarthritis, tendonitis, bursitis, MS and repetitive strain injuries.

Externally Gum ointment for boils, wounds and sores, psoriasis and urticaria. • Speeds healing of wounds and bruises, haemorrhoids and skin problems.

CAUTION Avoid during pregnancy. May cause mild gastric upset.

Calendula officinalis
Marigold

Native to Europe and Asia, this garden annual has been valued as a medicine since Roman times for digestive problems and infections.

Family Asteraceae

Parts used Flower

Actions Antiseptic, anti-inflammatory, diaphoretic, bitter tonic, digestive, antiulcer, antitumour, antioxidant, astringent, antiviral, detoxifying, antispasmodic, oestrogenic, diuretic.

Digestion Reduces inflammation in gastritis and peptic ulcers. • Astringent for diarrhoea and bleeding. • Bitters stimulate liver and gall bladder function. • Antimicrobial and anthelmintic for amoebic infections and worms, pelvic and bowel infections, dysentery, viral hepatitis and dysbiosis.

Circulation Improves venous return; relieves varicose veins. • Enhances circulation and brings blood to the periphery, helping to throw off toxins.

Musculoskeletal system Depurative and anti-inflammatory for rheumatism, arthritis and gout.

Immune system Antioxidant and free-radical scavenging effects may account for its antibacterial and anti-inflammatory properties. • Polysaccharides have immunostimulant properties, antibacterial and antiviral activity effective in flu and herpes viruses. • Reduces lymphatic congestion

Urinary system Antibacterial diuretic for infections and fluid retention.

Reproductive system Regulates menstruation and relieves menstrual cramps. • Relieves menopausal symptoms and reduces breast congestion. • Astringent for excessive menstrual bleeding and uterine congestion. • Promotes contractions in childbirth.

Externally Stops bleeding, prevents infection and speeds healing of cuts and abrasions and ulcers.

CAUTION Avoid during pregnancy.

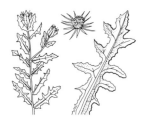
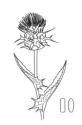

Cnicus benedictus
Holy thistle

This prickly annual with its yellow flowers is native to the Mediterranean. It has an ancient reputation as a digestive and liver remedy with the power to fight off malaria, smallpox and even the plague.

Family Asteraceae

Parts used Root, aerial parts, seed

Actions Diaphoretic, astringent, antimicrobial, digestive, carminative, decongestant, antispasmodic, stimulant, tonic, emmenagogue, expectorant.

Digestion Bitters enhance appetite, digestion and absorption, stimulate liver function and the flow of bile; used for anorexia, indigestion, wind, colic and conditions associated with a sluggish liver such as skin problems, headaches, lethargy and irritability. • Good astringent for diarrhoea.

Circulation Enhances the circulation and helpful for varicose veins.

Mental and emotional Nerve tonic, improves memory and relieves nerve pain, backache, headaches, migraines and dizziness.

Respiratory system Hot infusion is diaphoretic for fevers and expectorant for chest problems.

Immune system Excellent tonic after illness, when tired and run-down. • Enhances immunity and has an antimicrobial and antitumour action. • Taken hot it reduces fevers and catarrh and improves circulation.

Urinary system Diuretic; reduces fluid retention and cystitis.

Reproductive system Increases milk production. • Reduces heavy periods, menstrual headaches and period pain. • Emmenagogue; brings on suppressed periods. • Helpful during menopause.

Externally Antiseptic; staunches bleeding from cuts and speeds healing of wounds.

CAUTION Avoid during pregnancy

Carduus marianus
Milk thistle

Native to the Mediterranean and naturalized in North America, Europe and Asia, milk thistle gets its name from the milky-white patterning on its toothed leaves, which resembles spilt milk. It has been used for centuries to treat liver and gall bladder problems.

Family Asteraceae

Parts used Seed

Actions Anti-inflammatory, antidepressant, antioxidant, appetite stimulant, astringent, bitter tonic, cholagogue, demulcent, diaphoretic, digestive, diuretic, emmanagogue, hepatoprotective, stomachic, tonic.

Digestion Hepatoprotective for acute and chronic liver disease. Increases the resilience of healthy cells by preventing toxins entering liver cells and stimulates the repair of cells damaged by infection, alcohol and drug abuse, chemical exposure and drugs such as in chemotherapy. • Silymarin acts as an antioxidant, decreasing free radical damage in the liver. • Prevents fatal poisoning from liver damage from mushrooms such as death cap if administered intravenously within 48 hours. • Indicated in acute and chronic viral hepatitis, bile duct inflammation and cirrhosis. • Traditionally used for gallstones and improving appetite and digestion in patients with liver disease. • Reduces cholesterol. • Detoxifying; useful in skin problems such as psoriasis. • Laxative; relieves haemorrhoids.

Immune system Anti-inflammatory action. • Improves immunity by enhancing the function of neutrophils, T lymphocytes and leucocytes. • May have anticancer actions in inhibiting the growth of breast, cervical and prostate cancer cells. • Maintains gut flora; used to treat candida.

Urinary system Protective action on the kidneys, reducing damage caused by toxins and drugs.

Reproductive system Leaves traditionally used to enhance the flow of breast milk in lactating women.

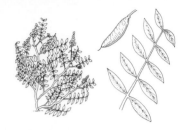
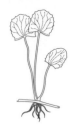

Cassia senna

Senna

This perennial herb with spikes of yellow flowers is native to North Africa, parts of the Middle East and southern India. Senna has been popular in the Arab world since at least the ninth century and is now famous throughout the world as a powerful laxative.

Family Caesalpiniaceae

Parts used Leaf, seed pod

Actions Cathartic, cholagogue, diuretic, febrifuge, laxative, purgative, stimulant, vermifuge.

Digestion Laxative; for acute constipation, flatulence and haemorrhoids, to soften the stool in haemorrhoids and anal fissures. Anthraquinones stimulate irritation and subsequent contraction of bowel muscle. It increases the flow of water and electrolytes into the large intestine and prevents fluid absorption, loosening and easing the passage of the stool. Best combined with aromatic herbs such as Ginger, Mint and Fennel, which relax intestinal muscles to prevent griping and improve bitter taste. • Antimicrobial for bowel infections. • Clears heat from the liver; indicated for jandice and liver problems. • Clears heat and toxins via the bowels; may be useful in fevers, arthritis and gout. • Anthelmintic action counteracts worms.

Circulation Used in Traditional Chinese Medicine to combat the build-up of cholesterol in arteries, clear heat from the liver and to benefit the eyes. • Used in Ayurvedic medicine for anaemia.

Immune system Contains emodin with antibacterial properties.

Skin Clears heat and toxins; for skin problems such as acne, fungal infections, spots and boils.

CAUTION For short-term use only. Avoid in pregnancy and lactation, with IBS and gastrointestinal inflammation.

Drug interactions Avoid with cardiac glycosides such as digoxin.

Centella asiatica

Gotu kola/Brahmi

This creeping annual native to Asia, Australia and the South Pacific is found in damp, marshy ground. Used traditionally to enhance memory and concentration, and promote intelligence.

Family Apiaceae

Parts used Aerial parts

Actions Nerve tonic, immunostimulant, febrifuge, alterative, diuretic, anthelmintic, rejuvenative, hair tonic, anticonvulsant, anxiolytic, analgesic, antibacterial, antiviral.

Digestion Used for indigestion, acidity and ulcers. • Antibacterial action contributes to its antiulcer properties.

Circulation Relieves oedema, venous insufficiency and varicose veins. • Excellent wound and scar healer. Stimulates synthesis of collagen and production of fibroblasts; protects skin against radiation. • Prevents bleeding; helpful for anaemia.

Mental and emotional Famous brain tonic; protects against ageing effects and Alzheimer's disease. • Improves memory and concentration; excellent for children with learning difficulties such as ADHD and mental problems, autism and Asperger syndrome. • Used for depletion by stress and anxiety, insomnia and depression; calms mental turbulence.

Immune system Antibacterial against pseudomonas and Streptococcus spp.; antiviral against herpes simplex. • Clears toxins and allays inflammation.

Skin Clears boils, acne and ulcers. • Keratinocyte antipoliferant for psoriasis. • Increases synthesis of collagen and fibronectin; speeds wound healing.

Externally Juice from fresh leaves mixed with Turmeric is applied to wounds to speed healing. • Prepared in coconut oil, it is applied to the head to calm the mind, promote sleep, and relieve headaches; applied to the skin for eczema and herpes.

Drug interactions Can potentiate the action of anxiolytics.

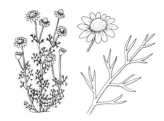
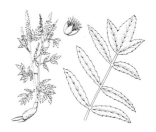

Chamomilla recutita

German and Roman chamomile

German chamomile is native to Europe and northern Asia; Roman chamomile is native to Europe. Both have sedative effects.

Family Asteraceae

Parts used Flowers

Actions Anti-inflammatory, antispasmodic, sedative, antiulcer, antihistamine, digestive, antimicrobial, diaphoretic, anodyne, diuretic, emmenagogue.

Digestion Soothes stress-related digestive upsets; relieves spasm, colic (particularly in babies), wind, indigestion, heartburn and acidity. • Bisabolol speeds the healing of ulcers. • Antimicrobial; resolves infections such as gastroenteritis.

Mental and emotional Calms anxiety and tension. Excellent relaxant for babies and children. • Promotes sleep and relieves pain in headaches, migraine, neuralgia, flu, arthritis and gout.

Respiratory system In warm tea it is used for fevers and infections such as sore throats, tonsillitis, colds and flu. • Reduces broncho-constriction in asthma.

Immune system Enhances immunity • Active against bacteria including Staphylococcus aureus and fungal infections including candida. • Antihistamine for allergies. • Reduces inflammation.

Urinary system Antiseptic diuretic; soothes inflamed/irritable bladder and cystitis.

Reproductive system Reduces period pain, PMS and premenstrual headaches. • Used for amenorrhea due to psychological problems. • For nausea and sickness in pregnancy. • Eases contractions and pain during childbirth. • Relieves mastitis. • Reduces menopausal symptoms.

Externally Stimulates tissue repair, speeds healing of ulcers, sores, burns, varicose ulcers and skin disorders. • Antiseptic wash for conjunctivitis; sitz bath for cystitis; and douche for vaginal infections

CAUTION May cause contact dermatitis.

Cimicifuga racemosa

Black cohosh

This perennial is native to North America and was renowned among Native Americans for easing mentrual problems and aiding childbirth.

Family Ranunculaceae

Parts used Dried root, rhizome

Actions Antispasmodic, anti-inflammatory, anodyne, hypoglycaemic, sedative, uterine tonic, diaphoretic.

Circulation Normalizes heart function. • Relaxes and dilates blood vessels; lowers blood pressure.

Mental and emotional Anemonin depresses the central nervous system; excellent for nerve and muscle pain, rheumatoid and osteoarthritis and headaches. • Eases cramps and muscle tension, ovarian and uterine pain, contractions during childbirth and breast pain. • Remedy for tinnitus and vertigo.

Respiratory system Antispasmodic; useful in asthma, whooping cough, paroxysmal coughing and bronchitis.

Musculoskeletal system Salicylates are anti-inflammatory, helpful in arthritis.

Reproductive system Regulates the menstrual cycle. Relieves PMS, breast pain and swelling, menstrual cramps and painful contractions in childbirth. • Taken several weeks before childbirth for safe and easy delivery. It has amphoteric action, relaxing uterine muscles when tense and toning them when weak. • Reduces heavy bleeding; strengthens uterine muscles. • Hugely popular for easing menopausal symptoms including anxiety, depression, hot flushes, night sweats, headaches, palpitations, dizziness, vaginal atrophy and low libido. • May normalize levels of luteinizing hormone and act on opiate receptors that affect mood, body temperature regulation and sex hormone levels.

CAUTION Avoid in pregnancy until last few weeks. It is an endangered species so only obtain from sustainable sources.

Drug interactions May interfere with oral contraceptives. Avoid with anticoagulant drugs.

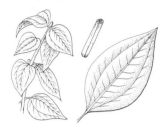
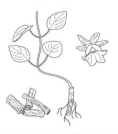

Cinnamomum zeylanicum
Cinnamon

C. zeylanicum grows in Sri Lanka. This sweet and aromatic spice, popular in cooking, is a warming remedy for warding off winter infections and improving digestion.

Family Lauraceae

Parts used Inner bark

Actions Antibacterial, antiviral, antifungal, antioxidant, tonic, immunostimulant, adaptogen, circulatory stimulant, antispasmodic, astringent, digestive, anaesthetic, probiotic.

Digestion Enhances digestion and absorption.
• Protects gut lining against irritation and infection, prevents inflammation and ulcers. Good for gastroenteritis and dysentery. • Combats candida.
• Enhances effectiveness of insulin; helps prevent glucose intolerance that can predispose to diabetes.

Circulation Lowers harmful cholesterol.

Mental and emotional Improves resistance to stress. • Lifts fatigue and low spirits, SAD and winter lethargy; used for chronic fatigue and ME.

Respiratory system Has a drying effect on mucosa.
• Expectorant for coughs and chest infections. • Decongestant inhalations used for colds and catarrh.

Musculoskeletal system Rich source of magnesium, essential for maintaining bone density. • Relieves arthritic pain, headaches and muscle stiffness.

Urinary system Antiseptic for bladder problems.

Reproductive system Helps maintain hormone balance. Good for PMS. • Uterine astringent, curbs heavy bleeding. • Aphrodisiac, used for low libido and impotence. • Used for painful periods.

Immune system Antiviral and antibacterial, helps throw off fevers. • Essential oil powerfully antibacterial, antiviral and antifungal. Inhibits growth of E. coli and Typhoid bacilli. • Combats thrush.

CAUTION Avoid large doses in pregnancy.

Codonopsis pilosula
Codonopsis

This perennial climbing herb native to Asia is famous as a tonic in Traditional Chinese Medicine, with properties similar to Ginseng.

Family Campanulaceae

Parts used Root

Actions Blood tonic, adaptogen, aphrodisiac, demulcent, depurative, digestive, emmenagogue, expectorant, immune tonic, hypotensive, kidney tonic, stimulant.

Digestion Improves digestion and assimilation. Promotes appetite, improves metabolism and aids weight loss. Used for weak digestion and diarrhoea.
• Calms hyperacidity and dyspepsia. Protects against gastritis and ulcers. • Reduces flatulence and nausea.

Circulation Dilates peripheral blood vessels, inhibits adrenal cortex activity, calms palpitations and lowers blood pressure. • Reduces blood-clotting processes and decreases risk of heart attacks and strokes.
• Increases red blood cell and haemoglobin count; benefits anaemia. • Invigorates the spleen, promotes the production of body fluid, improves the condition of the blood and curbs excessive sweating.

Mental and emotional Increases energy and enhances resilience to stress; used for debility and chronic fatigue.

Respiratory system Used for asthma, chronic coughs, shortness of breath, fevers and catarrh.

Musculoskeletal system Relieves rheumatic and joint pain. • Used to treat 'tired limbs', chronic fatigue syndrome and fibromyalgia.

Immune system Enhances the function of white blood cells and aids recovery from trauma, childbirth, surgery and illness. • Used for chronic immune deficiency, HIV and immune-suppressing effects of chemotherapy and radiotherapy.

Reproductive system Astringent properties reduce excessive uterine bleeding. • Strengthening to uterine muscles; prevents prolapse.

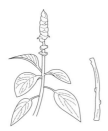

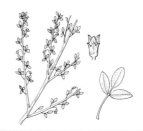

Coleus forskohlii
Forskohlii

This small perennial native to India, Sri Lanka and Nepal is used in Ayurveda as a heart tonic and remedy for the respiratory system.

Family Lamiaceae

Parts used Leaf, root

Actions Hypotensive, antiplatelet, bronchodilator, digestive stimulant, aromatic digestive, antiobesity.

Digestion Used for colic from muscular spasm.
• Enhances secretion of digestive enzymes.

Circulation Inhibits platelet activity, decreasing risk of blood clotting. • Increases force in heart muscle, improving heart function. Useful in angina and congestive heart failure. • Lowers blood pressure by dilating blood vessels.

Musculoskeletal system Antispasmodic for muscle tension and cramp, convulsions and bladder pain.

Immune system Immunomodulatory effect, activating macrophages and lymphocytes. • Useful in cancer management by inhibiting tumour metastases. • Reduces allergies and psoriasis associated with low cyclic adenosine monophosphate and high platelet activating factor (PAF) levels. Reduces histamine release and inhibits inflammatory response. • Excellent for asthma.

Endocrine system • Stimulates the release of thyroid hormone, relieving hypothyroid symptoms such as depression, fatigue, weight gain and dry skin.
• Increases fat metabolism and insulin production and improves energy. Popular for the management of obesity associated with low cyclic adenosine monophosphate.

Eyes Applied topically for glaucoma. Decreases intraocular pressure.

CAUTION Use with caution in hypotension and peptic ulcers.

Drug interactions Possible interaction with hypotensive and antiplatelet drugs.

Commiphora molmol
Myrrh

This tree is native to North Africa. When the bark is scored it releases a yellow oil that hardens into a resin, which is used medicinally.

Family Burseraceae

Parts used Oleogum resin (air-hardened gum resin)

Actions Astringent, antibacterial, anti-inflammatory, anthelmintic, lymphatic, antioxidant.

Digestion Protects the stomach lining from damage by drugs and alcohol. Heals peptic ulcers. • Combats worms and parasites.

Circulation Oleo-resins 'scrape' cholesterol out of the body. Used for congestive heart disorders, hypercholesterol and atherosclerosis. • Stimulates lymphatic circulation; reduces lymphatic congestion, inflammation, lymphoedema and lymphatic swellings.

Respiratory system Clears congestion. Used for fevers, chronic bronchitis, colds and catarrh.

Musculoskeletal system Anti-inflammatory for rheumatism and degenerative arthritis.

Immune system Increases white blood cells and antimicrobial against E. coli, Candida albicans and Staphylococcus aureus. • Sesquiterpenes are potent inhibitors of certain solid-tumour cancers.

Endocrine system Antioxidant, thyroid-stimulating and prostaglandin-inducing properties.

Reproductive system Stimulates circulation and moves stagnant blood; useful in amenorrhoea, endometriosis, fibroids, painful periods with clots, inflammation and congestion in the lower abdomen.

Externally Astringent and antibacterial mouthwash and gargle used for gingivitis, sore throats, aphthous ulcers, pharyngitis, tonsillitis and halitosis. • Speeds repair in cuts, wounds and slow-healing skin sores, bruises and broken bones.

CAUTION Avoid in pregnancy, excessive uterine bleeding and kidney problems.

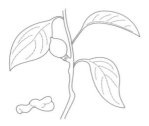

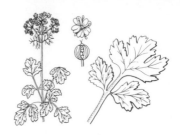

Commiphora mukul
Guggulu

This small tree is native to Asia and Africa. Its yellow resin is an honoured Ayurvedic remedy for 'scraping' toxins out of the body and lowering harmful cholesterol levels.

Family Burseraceae

Parts used Gum resin

Actions Anti-inflammatory, alterative, analgesic, antioxidant, antispasmodic, carminative, diaphoretic, expectorant, astringent, antiseptic, immunostimulant, rejuvenative, thyroid stimulant, emmenagogue.

Circulation Increases breakdown of LDL cholesterol and reduces triglycerides. Increases HDL cholesterol. • Inhibits platelet aggregation, prevents formation of clots and reduces atherosclerosis. Benefits ischaemic heart disease, angina and congestive heart failure.

Respiratory system Antimicrobial and antispasmodic for bronchitis and whooping cough.

Musculoskeletal system Anti-inflammatory and detoxifying for gout and arthritis. • Used for lumbago, rheumatism and sciatica. • Used for healing fractures.

Immune system Increases white blood cell count, clears infections and promotes immunity.

Endocrine system Specific for weight and obesity and hyperlipidemia, enhances thyroid function by improving iodine assimilation and regulates fat metabolism. • Can reduce blood sugar in diabetes.

Reproductive system Reduces accumulations in the lower abdomen. • Regulates the menstrual cycle.

Skin Reduces inflammation in chronic skin diease. • Helps regenerate tissue granulation and enhances healing. • Clears tumours and reduces lipomas.

CAUTION Avoid in acute kidney infections, excessive uterine bleeding, pregnancy and breast-feeding.

Drug interactions Can reduce the effect of antihypertensives; care needed with hypoglycaemic medication.

Coriandrum sativum
Coriander

This aromatic annual native to the Asia and the Mediterranean is valued in Ayurvedic medicine as a digestive and for cooling heat in the body.

Family Apiaceae

Parts used Seed, leaf

Actions Alterative, stimulant, carminative, diuretic, antibacterial, antioxidant, decongestant, antispasmodic, rejuvenative, aphrodisiac, digestive, refrigerant, analgesic, diaphoretic.

Digestion Enhances appetite, improves digestion and absorption. Useful in anorexia nervosa. • Relaxant and anti-inflammatory; relieves spasm, griping, wind, bloating, nausea, gastritis, heartburn, indigestion, nervous dyspepsia, halitosis, diarrhoea and dysentery.

Circulation Reduces harmful cholesterol.

Mental and emotional Invigorating and strengthening. • Clears the mind, improves memory, reduces anxiety and tension and promotes sleep. • Relieves headaches, migraine and other stress-related problems, muscle pain, rheumatism and neuralgia.

Respiratory system Seeds taken in hot teas for colds, flu, fevers, coughs and to ward off infection. • Decongestant for colds and catarrh, asthma and bronchial congestion.

Immune system Volatile oils in seeds are antibacterial and antifungal. • Fresh leaves used to chelate toxic metals from the body. • Brings out rash in eruptive infections such as chickenpox and measles.

Urinary system Diuretic; cools hot burning symptoms such as cystitis and urethritis. Reduces fluid retention.

Reproductive system Antispasmodic for period pain and uterine contractions during childbirth. • Aphrodisiac and energizing for low libido.

Externally Leaf juice/tea used internally and externally to soothe hot, itchy skin rashes. • Seed decoction used as a gargle for sore throats and oral thrush; eye lotion for conjuctivitis.

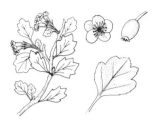

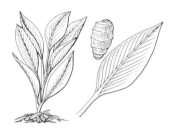

Crataegus monogyna
Hawthorn

This deciduous tree, is native to temperate climates. It provides excellent medicines for the heart and circulation.

Family Rosaceae

Parts used Flower, leaf, berry

Actions Antioxidant, hypotensive, circulatory stimulant, nutritive, rejuvenative, adaptogen, sedative, antibacterial, antispasmodic, astringent, digestive.

Digestion Used for diarrhoea, dysentery and dyspepsia. • Regulates metabolism.

Circulation Best remedy for heart and circulation, regulating blood pressure and preventing the build-up of atherosclerosis. Lowers harmful cholesterol. Strengthens heart muscle and regulates heart rhythm. • Prescribed in coronary insufficiency, palpitations, arrhythmias, angina and degenerative heart disease. • Protects heart muscle, reduces inflammation in blood vessels and helps prevent clots and heart attacks. • Peripheral vasodilator for poor circulation, Raynaud's disease and Buerger's disease, intermittent claudication and varicose veins. • Used for anaemia and altitude sickness.

Mental and emotional Relieves anxiety and stress; promotes sleep. • Recommended in ADD and ADHD.

Musculoskeletal system Benefits joint linings, synovial fluid, collagen, ligaments and vertebral discs. • Antioxidant for inflammatory connective tissue disorders. Useful in arthritis, gout and tendonitis.

Urinary system Diuretic; helps reduce fluid retention. • Dissolves stones and gravel.

Reproductive system Regulates blood flow; used for amenorrhoea. • Promotes libido and fertility. • Recommended in threatened miscarriage. • Used for menopausal night sweats and hot flushes.

Eyes • Used for macular degeneration.

CAUTION Drug interactions May potentiate effects of heart drugs such as digoxin amd beta-blockers.

Curcuma longa
Turmeric

This perennial native to South Asia has a long orange root that produces a yellow spice popular in Indian cooking.

Family Zingiberaceae

Parts used Rhizome

Actions Antioxidant, antibiotic, anti-inflammatory, digestive, analgesic, antiobesity, anticarcinogenic.

Digestion Aids digestion, absorption and metabolism. Aids weight loss. • Stimulates bile flow from liver, aids detoxification and protects the liver against damage. • Regulates intestinal flora; good after antibiotics. • Used for worms, heartburn, wind, bloating, colic and diarrhoea. • Soothes gut mucosa; boosts stomach defences against the effects of stress, excess acid, drugs and other irritants, reducing the risk of gastritis and ulcers.

Circulation Lowers harmful cholesterol and inhibits blood clotting by blocking prostaglandin production. • Helps prevent and remedy atherosclerosis.

Respiratory system Immune enhancing and antimicrobial; wards off colds, sore throats and fevers.

Immune system Enhances immunity. • Powerful antioxidant; protects against damage by free radicals. • Protects against cancer, especially of colon and breast. Enhances production of important cancer-fighting cells. • Curcumin is a powerful anti-inflammatory, excellent for arthritis, liver and gall bladder problems.

Externally Antibiotic and anti-inflammatory. Mixed with Aloe vera gel for inflamed and infected skin problems such as eczema, acne, psoriasis, scabies, fungal infestations and skin cancer.

CAUTION Avoid large doses in pregnancy and with peptic ulcers, obstruction of the biliary tract and gallstones.

Drug interactions Avoid large doses with anticoagulant and non-steroidal anti-inflammatory drugs.

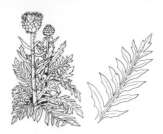

Cynara scolymus
Globe artichoke

The hardy perennial, indigenous to the Mediterranean region, is one of the oldest cultivated vegetables, valued by the ancient Greeks and Romans. It was used as a medicine by medieval Arab physicians mainly to treat the liver and sluggish digestion.

Family Asteraceae

Parts used Leaf

Actions Cholagogue, diuretic, antispasmodic, antioxidant, hepatoprotective, antioxidant, hypocholesterolaemic, astringent, detoxifier, digestive stimulant, diuretic, hypotensive.

Digestion Enhances digestion and absorption; stimulates metabolism. • Protective liver tonic, acts as an antioxidant, promotes regeneration of damaged liver cells and protects liver from damage from drugs, alcohol or chemicals. Often combined with Milk thistle, Turmeric or Schisandra for this and for hepatitis B and C. • Increases bile secretion and lowers harmful cholesterol. Indicated in liver and gall bladder disorders. • Anti-inflammatory and digestive action in the gut is useful in the treatment of Crohn's disease, IBS, dyspepisa, poor appetite, inability to digest fats, constipation and flatulence.

Circulation Protects the heart and arteries by lowering harmful cholesterol and lipid levels. Inhibits cholesterol synthesis.

Immune system Antioxidant; protects against free radical damage in cardiovascular system, immune system and liver. • 3,5 dicaffeoylquinic acid and 4,5 dicaffeoylquinic acid have demonstrated anti-inflammatory activity.

Urinary system Diuretic; relieves fluid retention. Aids elimination of toxins via the kidneys.

CAUTION Avoid in cases of obstruction in the biliary tract and gallstones.

Daucus carota
Wild carrot

This biennial is the ancestor of the domestic carrot. Native to Europe and parts of Asia, it is found in hedgerows and stony or sandy ground near the sea.

Family Apiaceae

Parts used Aerial parts, seed, root

Actions All parts: anthelmintic, astringent, carminative, diuretic, ophthalmic; seed: emmenagogue, abortifaecient, contraceptive, antitumour, spasmolytic, antifertility; root: antibacterial, liver tonic, urinary antiseptic.

Digestion All parts: improve appetite, digestion and absorption and expel worms from the intestines. • They relax the gut and relieve wind, bloating, colic and indigestion. • Stimulate the bile flow from the liver. Used for gallstones, sluggish liver and hangovers and to clear toxins. • May prevent damage to the liver from toxins, drugs and alcohol.

Immune system Cultivated carrots are rich in betacarotene, boosting immunity, helping to prevent degenerative disease and reducing the risk of cancer and heart disease.

Urinary system Seeds are particularly diuretic and dissolve stones and gravel. Used for fluid retention, cystitis, urethritis, prostatitis and bladder problems. • They aid elimination of toxins via the kidneys; helpful in gout and arthritis. • Root is more antiseptic for urinary tract infections.

Reproductive system Seeds traditionally used as a contraceptive. Research shows that they interfere with the implantation of fertilized eggs in the lining of the uterus and oil from the seeds may block synthesis of progesterone. • Root contains porphyrins, which stimulate pituitary gland and increase the secretion of female sex hormones.

Eyes Betacarotene enhances eyesight and night vision.

CAUTION Avoid seeds during pregnancy.

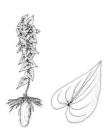

Dioscorea villosa
Wild yam

Wild yam is a creeping plant native to North and Central America. Until 1970 it was the sole source of the hormone material diosgenin, used in the contraceptive pill.

Family Dioscoreaceae

Parts used Root, rhizome

Actions Antispasmodic, anti-inflammatory, nutritive, rejuvenative, reproductive tonic, analgesic, antirheumatic, aphrodisiac, oestrogen-modulating, diuretic, cholagogue, relaxant, peripheral vasodilator.

Digestion Antispasmodic throughout the gut; relieves colic, spasms, IBS, biliary colic, painful wind and bloating. • Indicated in inflammatory conditions of the bowel such as colitis and diverticulitis.

Mental and emotional Calms anxiety, lifts depression and relaxes muscle tension.• Combats tiredness. • Relieves mood swings in PMS and menopause.

Musculoskeletal system Relieves muscular spasm and pain, muscle twitches and leg cramps. • Reduces inflammation; useful in arthritis and gout.

Immune system Anti-inflammatory, can be helpful in autoimmune disease such as rheumatoid arthritis and lupus.• Enhances immunity; may stimulate interferon production.

Reproductive system Regulates levels of oestrogen and progesterone; steroidal saponins are converted to diosgenin in the body, a precursor of progesterone. • Relieves tension and cramps in the uterus and ovaries; used for spasmodic dysmenorrhoea with nausea and ovarian pain. • Used for nausea and cramping in pregnancy, especially when related to stress and tension, and for threatened miscarriage. • Can be helpful for menopausal symptoms such as hot flushes, insomnia and night sweats.

Externally Used in creams to balance hormones and reduce menopausal symptoms.

CAUTION An ovredose may cause nausea, vomiting, diarrhoea and headache.

Echinacea angustifolia, purpurea,. pallida
Echinacea

This plant is native to North America. It was traditionally valued as a blood cleanser for wounds, burns, insect bites and joint pains.

Family Asteraceae

Parts used Whole herb, root

Actions Alterative, antibiotic, diaphoretic, antioxidant, anti-inflammatory, immunostimulant, antimicrobial, decongestant, antitumour, diaphoretic.

Respiratory system Wards off infections especially when taken at the onset of sore throats, colds, chest infections, tonsillitis and glandular fever. • Relieves chronic respiratory tract infections and whooping cough. • Traditionally used for TB.

Immune system Immune-stimulating; increases the activity of white blood cells. • Antibiotic, antifungal, antiviral and antiallergenic action. • Recommended for candida and post-viral fatigue syndrome. • Particularly useful for lowered immunity that causes repeated infections and antibiotic resistance. • Helps support immunity in cancer and after chemotherapy and radiotherapy. • The anti-inflammatory effect of Echinacea helps relieve arthritis and gout, skin conditions and pelvic inflammatory disease. • Taken in hot infusion it stimulates circulation and sweating, reducing fevers. • Traditionally used for malaria and typhus.

Reproductive system Indicated for gynaecological infections, pelvic inflammatory disease, urinary infections and post-partum infection.

Skin Blood cleanser for septic conditions; clears skin of infections, boils and abscesses. • Relieves allergies such as urticaria and eczema.

Externally Anti-inflammatory and antiseptic for skin problems. • Gargle and mouthwash used for sore throats and infected gums.

CAUTION Occasional sensitivity may cause anaphylaxis, asthma or urticaria.

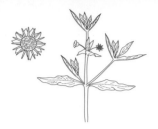
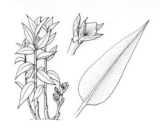

Eclipta alba
Bhringaraj

This herb has a daisy-like flower and is native to India where it is traditionally used to enhance memory and as an anti-ageing remedy. .

Family Asteraceae

Parts used Aerial parts, root, seed

Actions Antioxidant, alterative, purgative, antiseptic, antimicrobial, antiviral, rejuvenative, febrifuge, anti-inflammatory, haemostatic, anthelmintic.

Digestion Improves appetite, stimulates digestion and absorption. • Aids elimination of toxins by stimulating the bowels; indicated in constipation. • Excellent for liver problems including cirrhosis and infective hepatitis. • Protects liver against damage from drugs, chemicals and alcohol. • Acts as a deobstruent to promote bile flow. • Protects parenchymal liver tissue in viral hepatitis and other conditions involving liver enlargement.

Circulation Reduces blood pressure and nervous palpitations. • Used for anaemia.

Mental and emotional Valued in Ayurveda as a rejuvenative. Antioxidant properties reduce oxidative and ischaemic damage to the brain and improve brain function, memory and concentration. Prevents onset of age-related mental decline and Alzheimer' disease. • Calms nervous tension and anxiety; helpful in insomnia, mental agitation and anger. • Traditionally used for vertigo, dizziness, declining eyesight and hearing problems.

Respiratory system Combats upper respiratory infections and clears catarrhal congestion.

Skin Aids liver in its cleansing work. It is beneficial for skin problems including urticaria, eczema, psoriasis and vitiligo. • Reduces itching and inflammation; traditionally reputed to promote a lustrous complexion.

Externally Combined with coconut oil, it is a popular remedy for balding and premature hair greying by nourishing the roots.

Elettaria cardamomum
Cardamom

Native to India, aromatic and spicy Cardamom can neutralize the overstimulating effects of caffeine and reduce the mucous-forming properties of milk by aiding its digestion.

Family Zingiberaceae

Parts used Seed

Actions Carminative, antispasmodic, decongestant, expectorant, diaphoretic, digestive, circulatory stimulant, antibacterial, aphrodisiac.

Digestion Warming and invigorating, cardamom improves appetite, digestion and absorption and sweetens breath. • Seeds chewed or in teas are used for relaxing stress-related problems, indigestion, colic, wind, nausea, vomiting (including that related to chemotherapy) and travel sickness. Often combined with Fennel. • Counteracts excess acidity in the stomach • Prevents post-prandial drowsiness and hangovers from alcohol. • It has a mild laxative effect.

Circulation Enhances circulation and increases energy; good when run-down and tired in the winter.

Mental and emotional For tension and anxiety, lethargy and nervous exhaustion. • Lifts the spirits, calms the mind. • Improves memory and concentration.

Respiratory system Seeds chewed soothe sore throats and dry coughs. • Stimulating expectorant action clears phlegm from the nose, sinuses and chest in colds, coughs, asthma and chest infections.

Musculoskeletal system Essential oil is anti-inflammatory and analgesic for joint pain.
• Antispasmodic for muscle pain and spasm.

Urinary system Strengthening for a weak bladder, involuntary urination and bed-wetting in children.
• Antibacterial for urinary tract infections.
Reproductive system Traditionally used as an aphrodisiac and added to love potions.

CAUTION Avoid large amounts in cases of gastro-oesophageal reflux and gallstones.

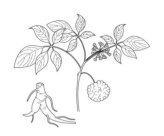
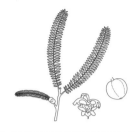

Eleutherococcus senticosus
Siberian ginseng

A famed tonic that grows in Siberia, China, Korea and Japan and long used for increasing vitality, improving mental and physical performance and protecting against stress.

Family Araliaceae

Parts used Root

Actions Adaptogen, antioxidant, immunostimulant, hypocholesterolaemic, anti-inflammatory, rejuvenative.

Digestion Improves digestion and absorption of nutrients, increasing strength and relieving lethargy, diarrhoea and bloating from weak digestion. • Protects the liver; enhances its ability to break down toxins. • Regulates blood sugar levels.

Circulation Reduces harmful cholesterol and triglycerides. • Relieves angina. • Relaxes arteries; reduces stress-related blood pressure. • Normalizes body temperature; helpful in hypothermia.

Mental and emotional Increases blood flow through the arteries to the brain; improves memory and concentration and increases mental stamina. Used for ADHD and failing memory in the elderly • Supports optimum adrenal function; useful for adrenal fatigue.

Musculoskeletal system Excellent for athletes. Powerful anti-fatigue effect; increases endurance and ability of the mitochondria in the cells to produce energy. • Increases cells' ability to dispose of lactic acid causing sore muscles after a workout.

Immune system Wide research in Russia on athletes and workers demonstrated its ability to help cope with and recover from adverse conditions and physical performance. • Enhances immunity against infections including coughs and colds, protects against carcinogens including environmental pollutants and radiation and inhibits tumour formation. • Speeds recovery after physical exertion; prevents immuno-depletion from excessive work.

CAUTION Drug interactions Avoid with digoxin.

Emblica officinalis
Amalaki/Indian gooseberry

Native to India, this fruit is one of the richest natural sources of vitamin C, containing approximately 20 times the vitamin C content of an orange.

Family Euphorbiaceae

Parts used Mainly fruit, to a lesser extent seed, leaf, root, bark, flower

Actions Rejuvenative, antioxidant, hepatoprotective, hypocholesterolaemic, anti-inflammatory, laxative, hypoglycaemic, stomachic, tonic, diuretic, antifungal.

Digestion Enhances appetite, digestion and absorption. • Antibacterial and anti-inflammatory properties helpful for peptic ulcers, acidity, nausea, vomiting, gastritis, hepatitis, colitis and haemorrhoids. • An ingredient of the cleansing formula Triphala. A bowel tonic for IBS and chronic constipation. • Antioxidant properties protect the liver.

Circulation Decreases LDH cholesterol levels; reduces atherosclerosis. • Reduces risk of blood clots.

Mental and emotional Famous rejuvenative for debility following illness, stress or in old age. Main ingredient of tonic Chayawanprash to improve mental and physical wellbeing. • Improves memory and concentration and resilience to stress. Calms anger.

Respiratory system Antibiotic activity against a wide range of bacteria; used for coughs, colds, flu, chest infections and asthma.

Immune system Shown to slow the growth of cancer cells, probably through its ability to enhance natural cell mediated cytotoxicity. • Antifungal; useful for candida. • Antiviral for colds and flu. • Active against a range of organisms including Staphylococcus aureus, E. coli, L. albicans, Mycobacterium tuberculosis and Staphylococcus typhos. • Antioxidant and immunomodulating.

Urinary system Antiseptic diuretic; resolves cystitis.

CAUTION Avoid in diarrhoea and dysentery.

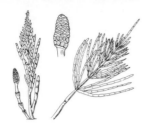
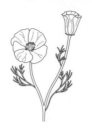

Equisetum arvense
Horsetail

Horsetail is a prehistoric-looking perennial and is one of the oldest plants on the planet. Native to Europe, Asia, Africa and North America, it is found growing wild in damp ground. It is highly valued as a rich source of minerals and trace elements.

Family Equisetaceae

Parts used Aerial parts

Actions Diuretic, antihaemorrhagic, alterative, anodyne, antibacterial, antifungal, anti-inflammatory, antiseptic, astringent, diaphoretic, kidney tonic, lithotriptic, nutritive, rejuvenative, tonic.

Digestion Astringent and toning useful for treating diarrhoea, rectal prolapse and haemorrhoids.

Circulation Stops bleeding of wounds, nosebleeds and in the respiratory and urinary tract. • Good tonic in anaemia. • Protects arteries from atherosclerosis.

Musculoskeletal system Rich in soluble silica, which is readily absorbed. Supports regeneration of bones, cartilage and other connective tissue; increases strength and elasticity. • Ability to increase bone density in post-menopausal women with osteoporosis. • Strengthening for teeth and brittle nails. • Used for rheumatic and arthritic problems.

Urinary system Used for cystitis, urethritis and urinary stones. • Beneficial in prostate problems, acute and chronic prostatitis and benign prostatic hyperplasia. • Astringent tannins stem bleeding and are toning for prolapse, urinary incontinence and bed-wetting in children.

Externally Stops bleeding and speeds healing of cuts and wounds. • Antiseptic and anti-inflammatory for skin problems.

CAUTION Horsetail breaks down vitamin B1. Take alongside B complex supplementation. Avoid in oedema.

Eschscholzia californica
California poppy

This vibrant yellow-orange flower is the state flower of California and native to western North America. It was first introduced to Europe as an ornamental and medicinal plant, but now has a reputation as a non-addictive alternative to the opium poppy for aiding sleep and reducing pain.

Family Papaveraceae

Parts used Whole fresh plant including root and seed pod.

Actions Sedative, hypnotic, antispasmodic, anodyne, febrifuge.

Digestion Antispasmodic, relaxes the muscles in the gut; relieves colic in the stomach and gall bladder.

Circulation By calming the nervous system it influences the heart and circulation; slows rapid heart, relieves palpitations and reduces blood pressure.

Mental and emotional Cousin to the opium poppy, but far less powerful. It is a safe sedative to calm excitability, restlessness, anxiety, tension and relieve insomnia; suitable for calming children. • Painkilling and relaxing for migraine, headaches, neuralgia, back and muscle pain, arthritis, sciatica and shingles. • Balances emotions and reduces stress. • Helpful in withdrawal from addiction to alcohol, drugs or tobacco. Helps to maintain mental stability. • Used for stress-related bed-wetting in children. • Beneficial for treating behavioural problems in children such as ADD and ADHD, improves memory and concentration.

Externally Applied to areas of pain such as toothache and headaches.

CAUTION Avoid in pregnancy and breastfeeding.

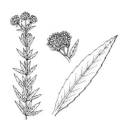
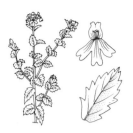

Eupatorium purpureum
Gravel root/Joe Pye weed

This handsome perennial with a mass of pink-purple flowers is native to Europe and North America and is found in moist woodland and by streams. Its common name is after Joe Pye, a New England medicine man who cured fevers and typhus with this plant.

Family Asteraceae

Parts used Rhizome, root

Actions Antirheumatic, astringent, carminative, diaphoretic, diuretic, emmenagogue, immunostimulant, tonic, alterative.

Immune system Used by Native American tribes as a diaphoretic to induce perspiration and reduce fevers.

Urinary system Diuretic, stimulant and astringent tonic to the urinary tract. • Reduces fluid retention. • Tea made from the roots and leaves drunk lukewarm to cool is used to prevent and treat kidney and bladder stones. • Reduces inflammation and soothes dysuria in cystitis, urethritis and prostatitis. • Helpful in treating arthritis and gout by increasing the elimination of uric acid and toxins via the kidneys. • Astringent action is helpful in treatment of urinary incontinence, bed-wetting in children and haematuria.

Reproductive system Tones and strengthens uterine muscles; stimulates contractions in childbirth. Recommended for threatened miscarriage and uterine prolapse. • Relieves menstrual pain. • Anti-inflammatory and astringent for pelvic inflammatory disease. • Indicated in benign prostatic hypertrophy and erectile dysfunction.

CAUTION Large doses may cause vomiting. Avoid during pregnancy. Contains pyrrolizidine alkaloids; do not take for more than 6 weeks.

Euphrasia officinalis
Eyebright

This delicate flowering annual is partially parasitic, taking nourishment from nearby grass roots. It is a member of the foxglove family, originally from Europe and Asia, but grows happily throughout the USA.

Family Scrophulariaceae

Parts used Aerial parts

Actions Astringent, digestive, liver tonic, alterative, demulcent, anti-inflammatory, expectorant, antibacterial, antiviral, antifungal, decongestant.

Digestion Bitters improve digestion and absorption and enhance bile flow, aiding the liver's detoxifying work and benefiting the eyes.

Mental and emotional Traditionally used to lift the spirits, for 'troubles of the mind' and to improve memory and concentration. • Regarded as a 'visionary herb', enhancing insight.

Respiratory system Astringent action relieves irritation and catarrh in nose, throat, sinuses, ears and chest. Used for sore throats, post-nasal drip, otitis media, sinusitis, sinus headaches and coughs. • Helps relieve allergic rhinitis/hay fever.

Eyes Used for centuries to improve and preserve eyesight. • Antimicrobial astringent for inflammatory eye infections such as conjunctivitis, styes, blepharitis and watery eye conditions. • Clears mucous, keeps eye mucosa clear and healthy. • Particularly used for red, itchy eyes with discharge, as in hay fever or measles. For oversensitive eyes that run in cold and wind and irritation from smoky/stuffy atmospheres. • Reduces inflammation in tired, strained eyes and puffiness. • Enhances circulation to the eyes; improves eyesight in the elderly.

Externally Gargles used for sore and catarrhal throats; mouthwashes for mouth ulcers. • To treat eye conditions it is best taken internally and used topically in sterile saline solutions as drops or compresses. • A few drops of dilute tincture or infusion in the nostrils used for clearing catarrhal congestion.

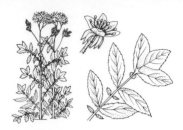
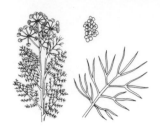

Filipendula ulmaria
Meadowsweet

These elegant flowers grow in damp meadows and by rivers and streams. When crushed they give off the characteristic smell of salicylicates, which offer similar benefits to aspirin.

Family Rosaceae

Parts used Aerial parts

Actions Analgesic, anodyne, antacid, antibacterial, antiemetic, anti-inflammatory, antispasmodic, astringent, cholagogue, diaphoretic, diuretic, relaxant, stomachic, urinary antiseptic.

Digestion Excellent antacid and anti-inflammatory for acid indigestion, heartburn, gastritis, peptic ulcers, gastro-oesophageal reflux and other inflammatory conditions. • Astringent tannins protect and heal the gut lining. • Antiseptic and antispasmodic; useful for enteritis and diarrhoea, IBS, colic, flatulence and distension.

Mental and emotional Analgesic for headaches and neuralgia. • Relaxant; eases spasm and induces sleep.

Musculoskeletal system Rich in vitamin C, iron, calcium, magnesium and silica. Speeds the healing of connective tissue. • Anti-inflammatory and analgesic; relieves pain and swelling in arthritis and gout.

Immune system Anti-inflammatory, analgesic and antipyretic activity; useful in acute infections, fevers, colds and flu. • Brings out rashes in eruptive infections such as measles and chickenpox.

Urinary system Mild antiseptic diuretic for cystitis and urethritis, fluid retention and kidney problems.
• Helps eliminate toxins and uric acid, which contribute to arthritis, gout and skin problems.

Externally Promotes tissue repair and staunches bleeding of cuts, wounds, ulcers and skin irritations.

CAUTION Salicylate sensitivity.

Drug interactions Possible interaction with anticoagulants. Do not take simultaneously with mineral supplements, thiamine or alkaloids.

Foeniculum vulgare
Fennel

This feathery perennial has large umbels of flowers that bear aniseed-tasting seeds. The Greeks used Fennel to overcome obesity and for stimulating milk flow in nursing mothers.

Family Apiaceae

Parts used Seed, leaf, root

Actions Anaesthetic, antibacterial, antiemetic, antifungal, anti-inflammatory, antispasmodic, antitussive, aperient, carminative, digestive, diuretic, expectorant, mucolytic, hormone balancing, stimulant.

Digestion Improves energy by enhancing appetite, digestion and absorption. Aids digestion of fatty foods. • Added to laxative blends to ease griping.
• Stabilizes blood sugar levels and reduces sugar craving. • Settles the stomach; relieves hiccups, colic, bloating, wind, nausea, vomiting, halitosis, indigestion, heartburn, diarrhoea and IBS. • Decongests the liver; clears stagnation.

Respiratory system Decongestant and expectorant in hot tea. • Relaxes the bronchi; useful in asthma.

Musculoskeletal system Diuretic action aids the elimination of toxins. This supports its anti-inflammatory effects in arthritis and gout.

Urinary system Aids elimination of toxins via the kidneys; used for cellulite, cystitis, fluid retention and urinary infections. • Helps dissolve stones.

Reproductive system Antispasmodic; relieves period pains. • Slightly oestrogenic. Regulates the menstrual cycle; used in amenorrhea, endometriosis, low libido and PMS. • Helpful during menopause.

Externally Decoction of seeds makes an anti-inflammatory eyewash for sore eyes and conjunctivitis, and a gargle for sore throats.

CAUTION Seeds are potentially toxic; do not exceed the recommended dose. In excess they can overstimulate the nervous system. Avoid therapeutic doses during pregnancy.

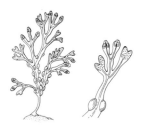
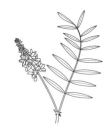

Fucus vesiculosus
Bladderwrack

A seaweed growing in offshore waters and temperate coastal parts of Europe and North America.

Family Fucaceae

Parts used Whole plant

Actions Antiobesity, thyroid stimulant, alterative, antimicrobial, anthelmintic, antioxidant, antitumour, demulcent, diuretic, emollient, laxative, nutritive.

Digestion Enhances energy as rich in nutrients. • Enhances digestion, mild laxative. • Probiotic for candida and intestinal worms. • Binds radioactive strontium, barium and cadmium in the gastrointestinal tract. • Relieves heartburn, gastritis and peptic ulcers.

Circulation Reduces harmful cholesterol levels through inhibition of bile acid absorption. • Reduces risk of heart disease, atherosclerosis, hypotension, hypertension and anaemia.

Musculoskeletal system Detoxifying, nourishing and anti-inflammatory for arthritic conditions.

Immune system Enhances immunity. • Contains the highest antioxidant activity of edible seaweeds; helps reduce cellular damage. • Antibacterial and antifungal properties. Polyphenols and polysaccharides have anti-viral and anti-inflammatory action; useful in herpes simplex and HIV activity.

Urinary system Diuretic; aids elimination of toxins. • Soothes inflammation in cystitis and urethritis.

Reproductive system Helps regulate the menstrual cycle. • Used to prevent breast cancer in Japan and can be helpful in fibrocystic breast disease.

Thyroid Used for low thyroid function and goitre. • Increases metabolism, demonstrating potential for controlling weight and cellulite.

CAUTION Avoid in hyperthyroidism, pregnancy and lactation.

Drug interactions Avoid with anticoagulants. Use with caution with insulin and antidiabetic drugs.

Galega officinalis
Goat's rue

This bushy plant with lilac blue flowers is an attractive perennial member of the pea family and is native to Europe, Russia and Iran. It was once important for treating the plague, fevers and infectious diseases and for treating diabetes mellitus.

Family Fabaceae

Parts used Aerial parts

Actions Hypoglycaemic, antidiabetic, diaphoretic, diuretic, digestive, antibacterial, febrifuge.

Digestion Galegine lowers blood sugar levels and helps manage late-onset diabetes. It contains guanidine, which reduces blood sugar by decreasing insulin resistance, helping cells to use insulin to metabolize glucose more efficiently. • Decreases absorption of glucose from the gut and reduces glucose formation in the liver; increases uptake and utilization of glucose in fat and muscle cells (metformin is a chemical derived from Goat's rue used to treat diabetes). • Helps non-insulin-dependent diabetics to regulate blood sugar levels and insulin-dependent diabetics to stabilize blood sugar levels and decrease insulin dosage. • Reduces appetite and increases weight loss; useful in metabolic syndrome X. • Enhances digestion and pancreatic function. Used for digestive problems caused by lack of digestive enzymes including constipation and indigestion.

Immune system Exhibits significant antibacterial activity against certain types of bacteria and inhibits blood clotting. • Diaphoretic; reduces fevers.

Urinary system Diuretic; reduces fluid retention and aids elimination of toxins via the kidneys.

Reproductive system Stimulates milk production in nursing mothers.

Externally Ointments are used to hasten healing after surgery.

Drug interactions Use with caution in patients on antidiabetic drugs or insulin.

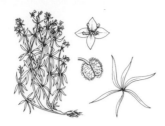
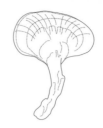

Galium aparine
Cleavers

This common hedgerow perennial native to Europe has long, sticky stems and seeds that cling to anything they touch. It is a member of the bedstraw family, so called because it was used as a strewing herb in less hygienic times, giving off a smell of newly mown hay.

Family Rubiaceae

Parts used Aerial parts

Actions Depurative, lymphatic, diuretic, aperient, tonic, astringent, anti-inflammatory, diaphoretic, cholagogue.

Digestion Improves digestion. • Stimulates bile flow from the liver. • May be helpful in hepatitis.

Circulation Lowers blood pressure, perhaps through its diuretic action. • Asperuloside may have hypotensive action.

Immune system Lymphatic tonic enhancing lymphatic circulation, aiding the body in its cleansing and immune work and purifying the blood. Recommended for lymphatic congestion, swollen lymph glands, glandular fever, ME and tonsillitis. • May have antitumour activity. • Clears heat and resolves inflammation; helpful in arthritis and gout. • Promotes immune function and reduces fevers.

Urinary system Diuretic; aids elimination of fluid toxins via the kidneys. Used for losing weight. • Traditionally used as tea or a vegetable as a cleansing 'spring tonic', cooling heat and clearing toxins. • Used for stones, urinary infections such as cystitis and irritable bladder.

Skin Cleansing for chronic skin disorders such as eczema, acne, boils, psoriasis and rosacea. • Helps resolve eruptive infections such as measles and chickenpox.

Externally Skin wash used for skin disorders, cuts and scrapes. • As a hair rinse for dandruff.

Ganoderma lucidum
Reishi

This mushroom grows on hardwoods in China, Japan, Russia and the USA. Known as the 'mushroom of immortality', Reishi was used for centuries as a longevity tonic.

Family Polyporaceae

Parts used Mushroom

Actions Tonic, immunostimulant, hypoglycaemic, antitumour, anti-inflammatory, antioxidant, expectorant, adrenal stimulant, radiation protective, cardio tonic, hypocholesterolaemic, antihistamine.

Circulation Enhances heart function and improves coronary artery circulation, protecting against heart attacks. • Relieves palpitations and arrhythmias, prevents clotting, normalizes blood pressure and prevents atherosclerosis. • Lowers cholesterol levels. • Increases oxygen level in the blood; used to combat altitude sickness.

Mental and emotional Reduces stress and anxiety. • Improves adrenal function and sleep quality.

Respiratory system Antihistamine action helps in allergic asthma and rhinitis. • Expectorant for chronic bronchitis, pneumonia and respiratory problems.

Immune system Beta-glucans enhance immunity and T-cell activity and increase production of leucocytes and macrophage activity; they protect against cancer. • Antibacterial to Staphylococci and Streptococci bacteria. • Antifungal; combats candida. • Used for HIV, herpes, hepatitis B and C, chronic fatigue syndrome, acute myeloid leukaemia and nasopharyngeal carcinomas. • Protects against the harmful effects of chemotherapy or radiotherapy. • Helpful in allergies; sulphur compounds inhibit histamine release from mast cells. • Gandosterone is hepatoprotective; beneficial for cirrhosis and hepatitis. • Excellent rejuvenative for the elderly and during convalescence.

CAUTION Avoid with mushroom allergies. May cause diarrhoea in large doses.

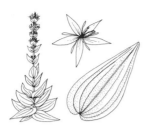

Gentiana lutea
Gentian

This beautiful perennial with yellow star-shaped blooms is found growing wild in lime-rich soil in the high altitudes of the European mountains. It has long been valued as a panacea for all ills and a vital ingredient of elixirs of life. It was used for stomach and bowel disorders, liver and heart problems, to neutralize poisons and to prolong life.

Family Gentianaceae

Parts used Root, rhizome

Actions Digestive, bitter tonic, anthelmintic, antiseptic, anti-inflammatory, antibiliary, emmenagogue, febrifuge.

Digestion The root contains the bitter glycoside amarogentin. Bitters stimulate the flow of digestive enzymes and stimulate appetite and digestion, particularly of protein and fats. • Aids absorption of essential minerals and vitamins and improves the elimination of wastes. • Stimulates bile flow from the liver. • Promotes peristalsis and movement of food and wastes through the gut. • Helpful in poor appetite, nausea, indigestion and wind. • Anti-inflammatory and cooling in gastritis and colitis. • Anthelmintic and antiseptic for clearing worms and infections.

Immune system Strengthening tonic due to its beneficial effect on digestion and absorption, which increases energy and immunity. • Traditionally used as a 'spring bitter' to purify the blood. • Anti-inflammatory, nourishing and cleansing. Relieves rheumatism, arthritis and gout. • Reduces fevers. • Gentiopicrin is highly poisonous to Plasmodium, accounting for its traditional use in treating malaria.

Reproductive system Emmenagogue; brings on periods and regulates menstruation. • Nerve tonic for PMS and menopausal mood swings.

Ginkgo biloba
Ginkgo

Native to China, this tree is popular for slowing the effects of ageing, such as poor memory, hearing loss and risk of stroke.

Family Ginkgoaceae

Parts used Leaf

Actions Antioxidant, circulatory stimulant, neuroprotective, antibacterial, anticoagulant, antifungal, anti-inflammatory, brain tonic, decongestant, kidney tonic, rejuvenative, vasodilator.

Circulation Improves blood flow and specifically cerebral circulation; protects against and treats altitude sickness, Alzheimer's disease, senile dementia and age-related poor memory, diminishing eyesight and hearing loss. • Indicated in impaired peripheral circulation, gangrene, Raynaud's syndrome and peripheral neuropathies. • Improves coronary circulation and relieves angina, arteriosclerosis and varicose veins. • Decreases blood viscosity; prevents clots. • Improves recovery in heart attacks, strokes and injury to the head.

Mental and emotional Relieves anxiety and depression.

Respiratory system Inhibits the activity of platelet-activating factors and inflammatory compounds associated with respiratory allergies such as asthma and chronic obstructive airways disease. • Enhances immunity to infections; helps prevent colds and coughs and chest infections.

Immune system Reported to have antitumour activity.

Eyes Protects the eye from damage by reducing free-radical damage to the retina. • Used for macular degeneration and impaired retinal blood flow. • Slows or prevents glaucoma, cataracts and diabetic retinopathy.

CAUTION Can cause headaches. Avoid a week before surgery and in haemophilia.

Drug interactions Avoid with anticoagulant drugs.

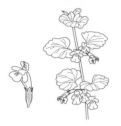
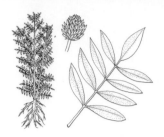

Glechoma hederacea
Ground ivy

Ground ivy is a creeping perennial with purple-blue flowers growing in profusion on grassland and in hedgerows and woods. Popular as a medicine since at least 2nd-century CE Greece, it has been used for treating inflamed eyes, chronic bronchitis and nervous headaches.

Family Lamiaceae

Parts used Aerial parts

Actions Anodyne, anti-inflammatory, appetizer, astringent, decongestant, digestive, diuretic, stimulant, tonic, expectorant, anthelmintic.

Digestion A pleasant-tasting digestive, enhancing appetite, digestion and the absorption of nutrients. • Protects the gut lining from irritation and inflammation and can be used for indigestion, wind, bloating, nausea and diarrhoea. • Traditionally used for expelling worms.

Respiratory system Astringent, antiseptic and decongestant; dries excess mucous in the nose, throat and chest. • Taken hot it makes a good decongestant for colds, catarrh, congestive headaches, coughs and bronchial phlegm, and helps to relieve fevers. • Safe and effective, it can be given to children to clear chronic catarrh and treat chronic conditions such as glue ear and sinusitis. • Traditional remedy for catarrhal deafness and tinnitus.

Urinary system Antiseptic diuretic; helps reduce fluid retention and clear toxins from the system. • Used for cystitis, urinary frequency and urinary tract infections.

Externally Used as a gargle for sore throats. • Makes a good lotion to bathe inflamed eyes and speed the healing of bruises, cuts and abrasions.

Glycyrrhiza glabra
Liquorice

This vetch-like perennial is native to Europe, Asia and North and South America. It has an affinity with the endocrine system.

Family Papilionaceae

Parts used Peeled root, runner

Actions Demulcent, expectorant, tonic, laxative, anti-inflammatory, antipyretic, diuretic, adaptogen, antacid, antitussive, adrenal tonic, antiviral, antiallergenic, hypocholesterolaemic.

Digestion Lowers stomach acid and relieves heartburn and indigestion. • Excellent for healing ulcers. • Mild laxative. • Increases bile flow from the liver. Useful in chronic hepatitis and cirrhosis.

Circulation Isoflavones reduce harmful cholesterol and atherosclerosis.

Mental and emotional Adaptogenic strengthening tonic. Improves resistance to physical and mental stress, possibly by its action on the adrenal glands.

Respiratory system Anti-inflammatory; soothes sore throats and dry coughs. • Expectorant for irritating coughs, asthma and chest infections. • Antiallergenic for hay fever, conjunctivitis and bronchial asthma.

Immune system Glycyrrhizin resembles adrenal hormones with anti-inflammatory and antiallergic effects similar (but without the side effects) to cortisone. Useful when coming off steroid drugs. • Antiviral; used for cytomegalovirus and herpes simplex. • Anti-inflammatory for arthritis, skin problems such as eczema and psoriasis.

Reproductive system Mild oestrogenic properties; used for menstrual and menopausal problems.

CAUTION Avoid prolonged use and large doses. May increase blood pressure. Avoid during pregnancy.

Drug interactions May cause potassium loss if combined with diuretics/laxatives. May potentiate prednisolone.

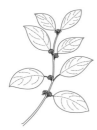

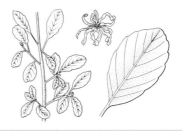

Gymnema sylvestre

Gymnema

This climbing vine, native to India and Australia, has been used for thousands of years in Ayurvedic medicine for balancing blood sugar. Its Sanskrit name gurmar means 'sweet destroyer' because eating fresh leaves numbs bitter and sweet receptors on the tongue.

Family Asclepiadaceae

Parts used Leaf

Actions Antidiabetic, astringent, diuretic, laxative, refrigerant, hypocholesterolaemic, hypolipidaemic, antiobesity.

Digestion Reduces sweet cravings and excessive appetite. Gymnemic acid binds to sugar receptors on the tongue for 1-2 hours, blocking the taste of sugar and reducing the desire for sweet foods. Helpful for weight loss. • Used in management of diabetes types 1 and 2, and blood sugar disorders. Increases production of insulin by the pancreas, helps to regulate blood glucose levels, helps the regeneration of beta cells in the pancreas that release insulin and stops adrenaline from stimulating the liver to produce glucose.

Circulation Saponins lower cholesterol and triglycerides.

CAUTION Saponins may cause or aggravate gastro-oesophageal reflux. Not to be used by patients with hypoglycaemia. Use with caution in heart conditions, as it can stimulate the heart.

Drug interactions In patients taking hyperglycaemic drugs and insulin, monitor blood sugar levels carefully so that the dosage of drugs can be adjusted.

Hamamelis virginiana

Witch hazel

This deciduous shrub, native to North America, has distinctive yellow flowers that appear before the leaves in early spring. Native Americans used it as snuff for nosebleeds and mixed it with flax seed for painful swellings and tumours. It is a household remedy for scalds and burns, to stop bleeding and bruising.

Family Hamamelidaceae

Parts used Leaf, bark, twig

Actions Astringent, haemostatic, slightly sedative, anodyne, antibacterial, anti-inflammatory, antioxidant.

Digestion Traditionally used for diarrhoea, dysentery, colitis and respiratory catarrh.

Reproductive system Astringent for uterine prolapse and a debilitated state after miscarriage and childbirth, as it tones up the uterine muscles.

Externally Tannins stop bleeding, speed healing, reduce pain, inflammation and swelling and provide a protective coating on cuts and wounds to inhibit the development of infection. It can be used in decoction, tincture or distilled form. As a douche for vaginal discharge and irritation; a gargle for sore throats, tonsillitis and laryngitis; and a mouthwash for mouth ulcers and bleeding gums. • Lotion can be applied to varicose veins, ulcers and phlebitis, insect bites and stings, aching muscles and broken capillaries. • Used as a poultice or compress for burns, inflammatory skin problems such as boils, swollen engorged breasts, bedsores, bruises, sprains and strains.• It makes a refreshing eyebath mixed with rosewater; relieves sore, tired or inflamed eyes such as conjunctivitis. • Potent antioxidant, used in antiageing skin preparations.

CAUTION Take internally only for short periods. Avoid in pregnancy and breast-feeding.

Drug interactions May impair the absorption of ephedrine, codeine, theophylline, atropine or pseudoephedrine taken internally.

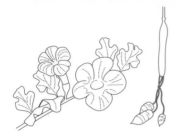
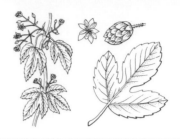
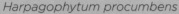

Harpagophytum procumbens
Devil's claw

This shrubby evergreen vine is native to the desert sands of Africa. It has been used by African tribes for hundreds of years to ease the pain of inflamed joints and clear toxins from the body.

Family Pedaliaceae

Parts used Root (secondary tuber)

Actions Anti-inflammatory, antirheumatic, analgesic, alterative, antibacterial, febrifuge, hypotensive, laxative, antispasmodic, bitter tonic, digestive.

Digestion Enhances appetite, improves digestion and absorption and eases stomach upsets. Useful in anorexia. • Bitter tonic for indigestion, flatulence, bloating and constipation.

Circulation May help lower both blood pressure and heart rate.

Musculoskeletal system Anti-inflammatory for arthritis, bursitis and tendonitis. • Used for degenerative disorders, osteoarthritis, rheumatoid arthritis, myalgia, lower back pain and gout. • Anodyne properties aid pain relief.

Externally Poultice can be applied to ulcers, boils and other skin lesions.

CAUTION Not advised in peptic ulcers, pregnancy and breast-feeding.

Drug interactions May interact with antiarrhythmic medications.

Humulus lupulus
Hops

A trailing plant that grows in Europe, Asia, North America and Australia. Hops used to be smoked for their narcotic effect, put in pillows for insomnia and used by monks to kerb sexual desire.

Family Cannabaceae

Parts used Female flowers (strobiles)

Actions Sedative, anaphrodisiac (male), bitter tonic, phytoestrogenic, antispasmodic, digestive, antiseptic, astringent, diuretic, anodyne, anti-inflammatory, antihistamine, expectorant, anthelmintic, febrifuge.

Digestion Bitters enhance appetite and digestion. • Eases muscle tension, spasm and inflammation; used for colic, IBS, diverticulitis, indigestion and stress-related problems including peptic ulcers, Crohn's disease and ulcerative colitis. • Tannins aid healing of irritated and inflammatory conditions and stem diarrhoea.

Mental and emotional Sedative and antispasmodic; relieves tension and anxiety as well as pain.

Respiratory system Antispasmodic, antimicrobial and expectorant; relieves coughs, chest infections, bronchitis and asthma.

Musculoskeletal system Anti-inflammatory and pain relieving for joint and muscle pain.

Urinary system Asparagin is a soothing diuretic • Aids elimination of toxins and helps clear skin problems such as eczema and acne.

Reproductive system Calms sexual desire in men and enhances it in women. • Reduces menstrual cramps. • Helps regulate periods and menopausal symptoms. • Enhances milk supply in nursing mothers.

Externally Add to a night-time bath to ease aching muscles and use in pillows to promote sleep.

CAUTION Avoid in depression. May cause contact dermatitis and stimulate oestrogen-positive tumours.

Drug interactions Avoid with central nervous system depressant drugs.

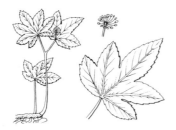

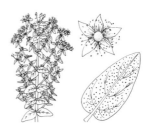

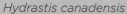

Hydrastis canadensis
Golden seal

This perennial woodland plant is native to North America and was a favourite of Native American tribes, including the Cherokees, Comanches and Iroquois. A powerful antimicrobial and anti-inflammatory, it has been used for ulcers, wounds and acute infections, including cholera, Giardia and amoebic dysentery.

Family Ranunculaceae

Parts used Rhizome, root

Actions Bitter tonic, anti-inflammatory, laxative, stomachic, anticancer, astringent, mucosal tonic, antimicrobial, antiseptic, antifungal, antispasmodic.

Digestion Improves appetite, digestion and absorption. • Relieves stomach upsets and indigestion. • Antimicrobial for gastroenteritis, diarrhoea and dysentery. • Probiotic; helps re-establish gut flora and combats candida. • Stimulates bile flow from the liver and helps the liver in its detoxifying work.

Circulation Enhances heart function and circulation; used in heart problems.

Immune system Stimulates the production of white blood cells to ward off infection. • Berberine has been found to be active against a wide range of bacteria, including Staphylococcus spp., Giardia and tapeworms. • Toxic to certain types of cancer cells. • Reduces fevers. • Used for sore throats, coughs, colds, catarrh, flu, chest infections and whooping cough.

Externally Drops used for inflamed eyes and earache. • Gargle used for sore throats; mouthwash for ulcers and inflamed gums.

CAUTION Avoid in pregnancy and with high blood pressure. This is an endgangered species, so only obtain it from sustainable sources.

Hypericum perforatum
St John's wort

This perennial blooms at midsummer. Its yellow flowers contain a red pigment believed to indicate its power to heal wounds and staunch bleeding.

Family Clusiaceae

Parts used Flowering top

Actions Antidepressant, anxiolytic, antimicrobial, antiviral, antineoplastic, antioxidant, anti-inflammatory, sedative, astringent, expectorant, diuretic.

Digestion Astringent and antimicrobial for gastroenteritis, diarrhoea and dysentery. • Heals peptic ulcers and gastritis. • Protects liver against toxins.

Circulation Reduces blood pressure and capillary fragility.

Mental and emotional Increases sensitivity to sunlight; reduces SAD during winter and jet lag. • Improves sleep and concentration. • Mood-elevating properties can take 2–3 months to produce a lasting effect. • Reduces nerve pain and neuralgia such as trigeminal neuralgia, sciatica, back pain, headaches, shingles and rheumatic pain.

Respiratory system Expectorant action clears phlegm; relieves coughs and chest infections.

Immune system Anti-inflammatory for gout and arthritis. • Hypericin has shown antitumour activity. • Antiviral; active against TB and influenza A, herpes, HIV and hepatitis B and C.

Reproductive system For painful, heavy and irregular periods, PMS and menopausal emotional problems.

Externally Oil eases pain and speeds healing in nerve pain such as sciatica and shingles, burns, cuts, varicose veins, ulcers, sunburn and inflammatory conditions.

CAUTION Can cause photosensitivity. Avoid during pregnancy.

Drug interactions Avoid with theophylline beta-2 agonists, SSRIs, protease inhibitors and cyclosporin.

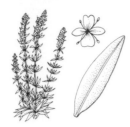
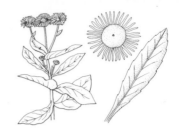

Hyssopus officinalis
Hyssop

This attractive evergreen member of the mint family is native to Europe and Asia. It was valued by the Romans as an effective antimicrobial remedy to protect against sickness, including the plague, and was used in the Middle Ages to clean churches and the houses of the sick.

Family Lamiaceae

Parts used Flower, leaf

Actions Expectorant, diaphoretic, diuretic, digestive, anthelmintic, antiviral, astringent, cholagogue, circulatory stimulant, decongestant, vasodilator, antiseptic, carminative, emmenagogue.

Digestion Increases appetite and digestion.
• Relieves indigestion, constipation and flatulence.
• Antispasmodic; reduces spasm, colic and IBS.

Circulation Pungent and warming; stimulates circulation, causes sweating, reduces fevers and increases the elimination of toxins via the skin.

Mental and emotional Traditionally used in epilepsy and as a cordial for the heart and to lift the spirits. • Nerve tonic to relieve anxiety, tension, exhaustion and depression, and give support during times of stress.

Respiratory system Stimulating decongestant and expectorant for colds, flu, catarrh, sinus problems, hay fever, coughs, asthma and pleurisy. • Volatile oils are antiseptic and expectorant; used for bronchitis, TB and viruses such as colds, flu and herpes simplex.

Immune system Excellent for warding off infection and enhancing immunity.

Externally Used as oils and liniments for bruises, sprains, cuts and wounds, aching joints and muscles, to relieve swelling and speed healing. • Oil in a vaporizer is used to purify the atmosphere, dispel infection, enhance clarity and concentration and steady the nerves when studying for exams. • Gargle used for tonsillitis and sore throats; inhalation for catarrh and hay fever.

CAUTION To be avoided by epileptics.

Inula helenium
Elecampane

This perennial with yellow daisy-like flowers is native to Europe and northern Asia. The bitter, aromatic root was traditionally used for children's coughs and catarrh.

Family Asteraceae

Parts used Root, rhizome

Actions Antimicrobial, expectorant, anti-inflammatory, analgesic, bitter, aromatic digestive, antispasmodic, bronchodilator, carminative, decongestant, anthelmintic, antibacterial, antifungal, emmenagogue, rejuvenative, diuretic.

Digestion Enhances appetite, digestion and absorption. • Relaxes tension and spasm and combats infection. • Calms nausea, indigestion, flatulence, colic, IBS, diarrhoea and gastroenteritis. • Stimulates bile flow from the liver. • Helps maintain healthy gut flora. • Alantolactone is active against roundworm, threadworm and hookworm infection.

Respiratory system A warming decongestant and expectorant, excellent for catarrh, colds, hay fever and bronchitis. Inulin is an expectorant. • Antispasmodic and antibacterial; used for sore throats, tonsilitis, laryngitis, whooping cough, asthma, emphysema, chest infections, pneumonia and pleurisy. Alantolactone has been found to be active against TB.

Immune system Enhances immunity and reduces inflammation; helpful in arthritis and autoimmune disease. • Antibacterial and antifungal; combats candida and dysbiosis. • Taken hot it helps to reduce fevers and increases circulation.

Urinary system Antiseptic diuretic; relieves fluid retention and urinary tract infections. • Antispasmodic for irritable bladder.

Externally Good antiseptic wash for cuts, wounds and skin infections such as scabies and herpes.
• Traditionally used for facial neuralgia and sciatica.

CAUTION Avoid during pregnancy. Large doses may cause diarrhoea, vomiting and allergic hypersensitivity.

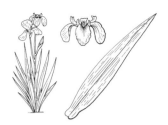
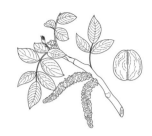

Iris versicolor
Blue flag

This perennial bog plant with purple-blue flowers is found growing wild in wet, peaty areas in North America and is the provincial flower of Quebec, Canada. It was popular among Native Americans as a remedy for skin diseases such as boils, abscesses and acne.

Family Iridiaceae

Parts used Dried rhizome

Actions Alterative, digestive, bitter tonic, diuretic, anti-inflammatory, cholagogue, diaphoretic, laxative.

Digestion Laxative, improves digestion and absorption, relieving flatulence, constipation, heartburn, indigestion and nausea. • Relieves headaches, skin problems and lethargy associated with poor digestion. • Improves liver and gall bladder function, aids the digestion of fats and enhances the detoxifying work of the liver.

Respiratory system Clears congestion in the chest, throat and nose. • Relieves swollen glands and sore throats. • Traditionally used in thyroid and pancreatic disorders.

Immune system Enhances lymphatic circulation and immunity. Used for swollen glands, chronic tonsillitis and lowered immunity. • Traditionally used to clear heat and toxins, as a cleansing and anti-inflammatory remedy for skin disease such as boils, abscesses, psoriasis, herpes and acne.

Urinary system Diuretic; aids the elimination of toxins and excess fluid via the urine.

Externally Root was used in poultices by Native Americans to relieve pain and swelling of sores, wounds, bruises and arthritic joints.

CAUTION The fresh root is poisonous. Only use the dried root in small amounts. Avoid during pregnancy and lactation.

Juglans regia
Walnut

This handsome tree, a native of Iran, grows happily throughout Asia and Europe. Walnut trees live a long time, some as much as 1,000 years. Many of the large trees seen in Europe and Britain were planted by monastic orders and in the grounds of convents for their nutritious nuts and the medicinal values of their leaves and green outer shell of the nuts.

Family Juglandaceae

Parts used Leaf, nut, bark, husks

Actions Alterative, astringent, anthelmintic, laxative, tonic, restorative, disinfectant.

Digestion Astringent action combats irritation and inflammation of the gut lining. Relieves indigestion, gastroenteritis, nausea and diarrhoea. • Traditionally used for worms and lowering blood sugar.

Respiratory system Clears catarrh and catarrhal coughs.

Immune system Walnuts are a good source of omega-3 essential fatty acids and linolenic acid, which benefits immunity and protects heart and circulation from degenerative disease. • Reduces harmful cholesterol. • Bark is detoxifying and enhances the function of the lymphatic system. Clears skin problems such as acne, lymphatic congestion and swollen glands.

Urinary system Diuretic and depurative action; aids elimination of toxins via the urine.

Externally Infusion/decoction of the leaves is used as a lotion for cold sores, shingles, chilblains, excessive perspiration of the hands and feet, piles, varicose veins and ulcers, inflammatory eye problems such as styes and sore throats. • Used as a douche for vaginal discharges. • Husks boiled in water are used as a hair dye (to cover up grey hair) and to thicken the hair. • The vinegar from pickled young walnuts can be used as a gargle for sore throats.

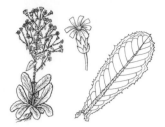

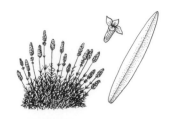

Lactuca virosa
Wild lettuce

This is the more bitter wild ancestor of the cultivated lettuce, native to North America, Europe and Asia. Its Latin name derives from lac, meaning 'milk', because of the white latex that exudes from the fresh stem, which has narcotic and euphoric properties. Dried leaves were traditionally smoked for relaxation and to relieve pain.

Family Asteraceae

Parts used Leaf, latex

Actions Sedative, antispasmodic, anodyne, narcotic, antitussive, diuretic, febrifuge, anaphrodisiac, bitter, digestive, cholagogue, hypoglycaemic.

Digestion Bitters stimulate bile flow from the liver; aid the elimination of toxins and the digestion of fats. • Used for nausea, indigestion, colic, pain and stress-related digestive problems.

Mental and emotional Alkaloids have a narcotic and euphoric effect similar to opium in large amounts, but not addictive. Calming for anxiety, panic attacks, hyperactivity, restlessness and agitation. Great sedative for inducing sleep. • Antispasmodic and analgesic; relieves pain and tension in tight muscles.

Respiratory system Antispasmodic and sedative to the cough reflex; calms dry, irritating coughs, particularly those that disturb sleep. • Used for bronchitis and whooping cough.

Externally Cooling wash used for inflammatory skin problems such as acne, spots and rash from poison ivy. • Latex is used to treat warts, applied daily.

CAUTION Can cause drowsiness if used during the day or in large doses. Latex from the fresh plant can cause eye irritation and rashes.

Lavandula spp.
Lavender

Native to the Mediterranean, this perennial shrub was popular during the Middle Ages as a strewing herb to perfume and sanitize houses and churches, and to ward off the plague.

Family Lamiaceae

Parts used Flower

Actions Carminative, diuretic, antispasmodic, nerve tonic, analgesic, stimulant, digestive, sedative, antimicrobial, antiseptic, diaphoretic, expectorant, antidepressant, antioxidant.

Digestion Releases spasm and colic and combats wind and bowel problems related to tension and anxiety. • Volatile oils active against bacteria and fungi. Used for infections causing vomiting and diarrhoea.

Mental and emotional Excellent for anxiety and stress-related symptoms such as headaches, migraines, neuralgia, palpitations, insomnia. • Helpful in agitated behaviour in dementia. • Lifts the spirits. • Restores energy in tiredness and nervous exhaustion.

Respiratory system Antimicrobial; increases resistance to colds, coughs, chest infections, flu, tonsillitis and laryngitis. • Decongesting and expectorant; clears phlegm and relieves asthma. • Antispasmodic for asthma and croup.

Immune system Volatile oils are antibacterial, antifungal and antiseptic. • Rosmarinic acid has antioxidant and anti-inflammatory action. • Taken as hot tea it reduces fevers and increases the elimination of toxins via the skin and urine.

Reproductive system Analgesic and antiseptic; used in baths to speed healing after childbirth.

Externally Antiseptic for inflammatory and infective skin problems such as eczema, acne, varicose ulcers and nappy rash. • Stimulates tissue repair; minimizes scar formation when oil is applied neat to burns, cuts and wounds, sores and ulcers. • Oil repels insects and relieves bites and stings, soothes pain of bruises, sprains, gout, arthritis and muscle tension.

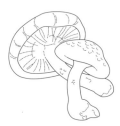
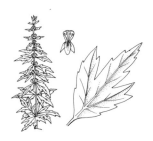

Lentinula edodes
Shiitake mushroom

This delicious edible mushroom is native to China. It has been used to prevent premature ageing for thousands of years.

Family Polyporaceae

Parts used Mushroom

Actions Immunostimulant, rejuvenative, antitumour, antioxidant, antiviral, aphrodisiac, hepatoprotective, hypocholesterolaemic, hypotensive.

Digestion Protects the liver against damage from toxins, chemicals, alcohol, drugs and infection. Can reduce elevated liver enzymes. • Regulates blood sugar.

Circulation Reduces cholesterol, blood pressure and atherosclerosis. Prevents clots. • Antioxidant action helps prevent cardiovascular disease, strokes and heart attacks. • Strengthening tonic for anaemia.

Respiratory system Boosts interferon production, which fights flu viruses. Enhances immunity; prevents frequent colds and coughs and bronchitis.

Immune system Powerful natural immunostimulant and restorative. Strengthens immunity of patients with cancer, HIV and TB, autoimmune disease, chronic fatigue syndrome and fibromyalgia. • Used for allergies, arthritis, environmental illness, fatigue and hepatitis. • Compound in cooked Shiitake (thiazolidine-4-carboxylic acid) can inhibit the formation of potentially carcinogenic nitrites in the stomach. • Lentinan can improve survival times of cancer patients when used concurrently with chemotherapy. • Stimulates stem cells in bone marrow to produce B and T cells; inhibits blood platelet aggregation and boosts production of interferon and natural killer cells, which help suppress tumours.

CAUTION Avoid in extreme weakness or with diarrhoea. Rarely causes mild gastric upset and rashes.

Drug interactions Thyroxin and hydrocortisone inhibit the antitumour activity of lentinan. Water-soluble extracts may reduce platelet coagulation; use cautiously with blood thinners.

Leonurus cardiaca
Motherwort

This perennial is found growing in hedgerows in many parts of Europe. It has been praised since the days of the ancient Greeks as a relaxing remedy for expectant mothers, hence its name.

Family Lamiaceae

Parts used Aerial parts

Actions Antispasmodic, anxiolytic, hypotensive, diaphoretic, astringent, bitter, partus praeparator, parturient, emmenagogue, thymoleptic, immunostimulant, antiviral, antibacterial.

Digestion Bitter and cooling for acidity and heartburn. • Antispasmodic for stress-related digestive problems.

Circulation Benefits the heart; reduces palpitations and blood pressure. • Reduces blood clotting, harmful cholesterol and atherosclerosis.

Mental and emotional Calms anxiety and aids sleep. • Reduces nervous palpitations and irregular heart rates, particularly useful during menopause. • Relieves headaches and muscular twitches and spasms.

Immune system Active against viruses such as Epstein Barr, herpes and bacterial and fungal infection. • Ursolic acid has been found to inhibit cancers including leukaemia and lung, breast and colon cancer.

Reproductive system Antispasmodic and tonic; for painful or delayed periods, cramps, back pain and vaginismus. • Enhances fertility, increases libido. • Helps prepare for childbirth, taken in the last few weeks; eases tension or anxiety about birth. • Eases childbirth. • Helps prevent post-partum infection. • Helps prevent post-natal depression. • Stimulates menstruation. • Soothes anxiety, anger and irritability; good for PMS and menopausal mood swings. • Helpful in menstrual headaches. • Cooling for hot flushes.

Externally Used as a douche/lotion for leucorrhoea and vaginal infection such as candida.

CAUTION May increase menstrual flow. Use only in the last few weeks of pregnancy.

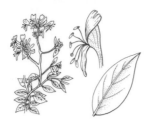

Lonicera japonica
Honeysuckle

This woody, deciduous twining shrub is loved for its honey-sweet scent. A syrup of the flowers is a traditional remedy for croup, cramps and asthma.

Family Caprifoliaceae

Parts used Aerial parts

Constituents Essential oils (including borneol), mucilage, glucoside, salicylic acid, invertin.

Actions Antimicrobial, antiseptic, rejuvenative, alterative, laxative, expectorant, astringent, diaphoretic, diuretic, hypotensive, antispasmodic, anti-inflammatory, decongestant.

Digestion Gentle laxative. • Anti-inflammatory and antiseptic; useful for diarrhoea, dysentery, food poisoning and Crohn's disease.

Respiratory system Anti-inflammatory, expectorant, decongestant, antibiotic and antispasmodic properties; useful for spasm and phlegm in asthma, croup, whooping cough, bronchitis and chest infections. • Active against several bacteria including TB. • The Japanese use flowers for sore throats, colds, flu, tonsillitis, bronchitis and pneumonia. • In hot infusion used for colds, catarrh, sinusitis and bronchial congestion.

Immune system Enhances immunity; promotes longevity. • Essential oils are antimicrobial; active against several bacteria and enhance the system's fight against infection. • Salicylic acid has an aspirin-like action, relieving aches and pains, headaches, flu, fevers, arthritis and rheumatism.

Urinary system Diuretic; soothing in cystitis and irritable bladder. • Aids elimination of toxins.

Skin Detoxifying and anti-inflammatory; clears spots, boils, acne, psoriasis and eczema.

Externally Lotion soothes rashes and sore eyes. • Gargle for sore throats; mouthwash for mouth ulcers.

CAUTION The berries are poisonous.

Marrubium vulgare
White horehound

A perennial native to Europe, Asia and North Africa, with woolly, silvery-green leaves and a musky aroma loved by bees. Popular in brewing, White horehound used to be made into sweets for catarrh and coughs.

Family Lamiaceae

Parts used Aerial parts

Constituents Flavonoids (luteolin), saponins, tannins, volatile oils (pinene, limonene and campene), mucilage, bitter lactone, alkaloids (betonicine and stachydrine), sterols, diterpene alcohol (marrubiol), bitters, vitamin C, iron.

Actions Expectorant, decongestant, diaphoretic, bitter tonic, anthelmintic, antibacterial, cholagogue, digestive, antispasmodic, diuretic, emmenagogue, laxative.

Digestion Its bitter taste stimulates appetite and digestion; promotes flow of digestive juices and bile from the liver. • Laxative. • Antibacterial and anthelmintic. • Indicated in indigestion, wind, colic, gastroenteritis, diarrhoea and worms.

Circulation Used for calming palpitations, dilating the arteries and normalizing the circulation. Essential oils have a vasodilatory action. • Contains iron; used for anaemia.

Respiratory system Renowned as an antibacterial, antispasmodic and expectorant remedy for coughs, colds, catarrh, flu, croup, asthma, bronchitis, chest infections, emphysema and bronchial catarrh. • Traditionally used for laryngitis, tonsillitis, pneumonia, TB and whooping cough. • Taken hot it increases perspiration and relieves fevers and catarrhal congestion.

Reproductive system Stimulates the uterus; brings on menstruation in delayed periods and amenorrhoea. • Traditionally used to expel placenta after childbirth.

CAUTION Avoid in pregnancy. Fresh juice may cause skin irritation.

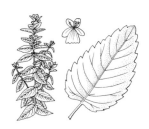
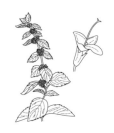

Melissa officinalis
Lemon balm

This perennial herb, native to the Mediterranean, was introduced to Britain by the Romans, who valued it to improve memory and lift the spirits. It was a favourite of the Arab world in the Middle Ages to promote longevity.

Family Lamiaceae

Parts used Aerial Parts

Actions Diaphoretic, carminative, antispasmodic, antihistamine, antimicrobial, sedative, antiviral, partus praeparator, antioxidant, decongestant.

Digestion Reduces pain and spasm. • Soothes stress-related problems. • Stimulates liver and gall bladder.

Circulation Calms nervous palpitations and arrhythmias. • Reduces hypertension.

Mental and emotional Sedative and analgesic; reduces tension, anxiety and agitation. Useful in dementia and insomnia. • Relieves headaches, migraine, vertigo and tinnitus. • Mood elevating. • Improves memory and concentration.

Respiratory system Relaxant, antimicrobial and decongestant; helps resolve colds, flu, catarrh, chest infections, coughs and asthma.

Immune system Antiviral against herpes simplex, mumps, possibly HIV. • Volatile oils are antibacterial, antifungal and antihistamine; helpful in hay fever and allergic rhinitis. • Rosmarinic acid is antioxidant and anti-inflammatory and influences complement activity.

Urinary system Antispasmodic and diuretic.

Reproductive system Helpful in irregular and painful periods, PMS and menopausal depression.

Externally Antiseptic for cuts and wounds. • Dilute oils used in massage for period pains, neuralgia, joint and muscle pain and cold sores. • Eardrops used for infections.

Drug interactions Avoid with thyroid drugs.

Mentha piperita
Peppermint

With its refreshing taste and stimulating action, Peppermint is used as a digestive, analgesic and decongestant for headaches and colds.

Family Lamiaceae

Parts used Aerial parts

Actions Diaphoretic, carminative, antispasmodic, antiemetic, antiseptic, digestive, circulatory stimulant, analgesic, antimicrobial.

Digestion Relieves pain and spasm in stomachaches, colic, flatulence, heartburn, indigestion, hiccups, constipation, IBS and diarrhoea. • Enhances appetite and digestion. • Relieves nausea and travel sickness. • Tannins protect gut lining from irritation and infection; useful in Crohn's disease and ulcerative colitis. • Bitters stimulate liver and gall bladder function.

Circulation In warm infusion it improves circulation, and causes sweating.

Mental and emotional Analgesic and antispasmodic; relieves tension headaches, joint and muscle pain.

Respiratory system Decongestant in hot infusion. • Clears airways and reduces spasm in asthma. • Enhances resistance to infections. Relieves colds, flu and fevers.

Immune system Increases energy and immunity by enhancing digestion and absorption. • Volatile oils are antibacterial, antiparasitic, antiviral and antifungal. • Active against a wide range of bacteria including Helicobacter pylori, Salmonella enteritidis and E. coli and fungi including candida.

Reproductive system Relaxes smooth muscle in the uterus; reduces menstrual pain and cramps.

Externally Oil used as an inhalant for colds, catarrh and sinusitis; added to lotions for muscular pains. • Tea/tincture used as a gargle for sore throats; mouthwash for gum infections and mouth ulcers.

CAUTION Oil should be used diluted, and avoided in pregnancy. Do not use on babies or small children.

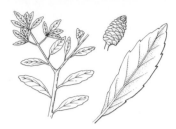
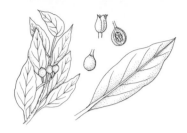

Myrica cerifera
Bayberry

This perennial shrub is native to eastern North America. The greenish berries are edible and produce wax that has long been used to make candles and soap.

Family Myricaceae

Parts used Bark, root bark

Actions Astringent, alterative, anti-inflammatory, antibacterial, antioxidant, circulatory stimulant, diuretic, diaphoretic, expectorant, hepatoprotective.

Digestion Astringent tannins protect the gut lining from irritation and inflammation. • Antibacterial actions also help combat infections. • Useful in gastritis, heartburn, acid indigestion, gastroenteritis, diarrhoea, dysentery, colitis and IBS.

Circulation Stimulates the flow of blood and lymph, clearing lymphatic congestion and supporting the detoxification work of the lymphatic system. • Used for varicose veins.

Respiratory system Astringes mucous membranes, protecting against irritation and infection and reducing excess mucous. • It has expectorant properties and brings down fevers. • Useful in colds, nasal congestion, catarrhal coughs, flu, sinusitis, sore throats and tonsillitis.

Urinary system Astringent diuretic, reducing fluid retention; recommended in urinary incontinence and bed-wetting.

Reproductive system Reduces blood flow; used for heavy periods. • Tones pelvic muscles; excellent for prolapse.

Externally Mouthwash used for bleeding gums and mouth ulcers, gargle for sore throats, and lotion for varicose veins. • Decoction used as a douche for vaginal discharge and combating infection. • Used in tooth powders for bleeding gums.

CAUTION Avoid during pregnancy.

Myristica fragrans
Nutmeg

Nutmeg is the dried kernel of the seeds of an evergreen tree native to the Indonesian Molucca Islands. It has long been used in love potions as well as perfumes and incense.

Family Myristicaceae

Parts used Kernel

Actions Sedative, euphoric, stimulant, anti-inflammatory, antimicrobial, antispasmodic, digestive, carminative, aphrodisiac, circulatory stimulant, astringent.

Digestion Relaxes muscles throughout the gut, stimulates the flow of digestive enzymes and promotes appetite, digestion and absorption. Relieves halitosis, indigestion, hiccups, colic, wind, bloating and nervous digestive problems. • Anti-inflammatory and antiseptic for Crohn's disease, colitis, infections, diarrhoea, dysentery, gastroenteritis, nausea and vomiting. • Traditionally used with coconut water in India for dehydration caused by vomiting and diarrhoea, particularly in cholera.

Circulation Protective effect on the cardiovascular system. Lowers harmful cholesterol. Prevents clotting.

Mental and emotional Powerful brain stimulant yet promotes sleep. • Relaxes muscles; eases muscle spasm and pain.

Respiratory system Decongestant for catarrh.

Reproductive system Traditionally used to prolong lovemaking and heighten sensitivity.

Externally Ground nutmeg mixed with water is applied to skin problems such as ringworm and eczema. • Essential oil can be applied to numb toothache while awaiting dental help. • The oil is anti-inflammatory and pain relieving used in rubs for arthritis, nerve and muscle pain.

CAUTION No more than 3 g should be taken daily. Large amounts can produce toxic symptoms such as nausea, vomiting, convulsions, tachycardia, restlessness, dizziness and hallucinations.

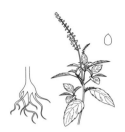
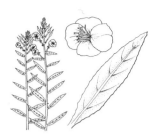

Ocimum sanctum
Holy basil/Tulsi

Tulsi has an uplifting and strengthening effect on mind and body. Its aroma is traditionally used to purify the atmosphere.

Family Lamiaceae

Parts used Leaf, seed, root

Actions Demulcent, antibacterial, antifungal, expectorant, anticatarrhal, antispasmodic, anthelmintic, febrifuge, immunostimulant, laxative.

Digestion Antispasmodic and warming; relieves spasm, wind and bloating. • Appetizing and digestive and improves absorption. • Used for anorexia, nausea, constipation, vomiting, abdominal pain, ulcers and worms. • Increases the production of protective stomach mucous, preventing irritation from acidity drugs and toxins.

Mental and emotional Uplifting and strengthening. Clears lethargy and congestion that dampen the spirits and fog the mind. • Reduces anxiety, mild depression, insomnia, and stress-related problems such as headaches and IBS. • Increases resilience to stress.

Respiratory system Decongestant, expectorant and antispasmodic. • Protects against histamine-induced bronchospasm; helpful in asthma and rhinitis. • Active against micro-organisms including E. coli, Staphylococcus aureus and Mycoplasma tuberculosis and fungi such as Aspergillus spp. • Used for coughs, colds, fevers, sore throats and flu.

Immune system Anti-inflammatory; inhibits prostaglandin production. • Protects healthy cells from the toxicity of radiation and chemotherapy. • Used for allergies such as hay fever and rhinitis. • Anthelmintic; active against enteric pathogens and candida.

Urinary system Relieves dysuria, cystitis and urinary tract infections. Clears toxins through diuretic effect.

Endocrine system • Lowers blood sugar, harmful cholesterol and triglyceride levels.

CAUTION Avoid during pregnancy.

Oenothera biennis
Evening primrose

This biennial was originally brought to Europe from North and South America. The oil is a good source of omega-6 fatty acids, vital for the healthy functioning of the immune, nervous and hormonal systems.

Family Onagraceae

Parts used Oil from seeds

Actions Antispasmodic, astringent, sedative.

Digestion Counteracts the effects of alcoholic poisoning; encourages regeneration of damaged liver. Helps withdrawal from alcohol.

Circulation Reduces high blood pressure and harmful cholesterol levels; helps prevent blood clots and coronary artery disease.

Mental and emotional Mildly sedative effect; good remedy for nervous indigestion and colic and hyperactivity in children. • Well known in the last few decades for its beneficial use in MS.

Respiratory system Can be used to relieve asthma and paroxysmal coughing, as in whooping cough.

Immune system Fatty acids are helpful in the treatment of allergies such as eczema, hyperactivity, ADHD, asthma, migraine, metabolic disorders, diabetes, high cholesterol, viral infections and arthritis. • GLA reduces inflammation by reducing prostaglandin E. • May enhance the production of free radicals and slow tumour growth.

Reproductive system Fatty acids help maintain hormone balance. Indicated in PMS, breast problems, menopausal problems and acne. • Increases fat content of breast milk when lactating.

Skin Provides GLA, which cannot be produced by the body; excellent when breakdown in GLA production from linoleic acid is related to problems such as eczema and acne.

CAUTION Avoid in epilepsy. Supplement with omega-3 oils simultaneously at ratio of 3:1.

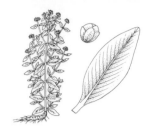

Olea europaea

Olive

The Olive is one of the oldest cultivated plants of the Mediterranean, thought to have been grown at least 5,000 years ago in Egypt and Crete for its oil.

Family Oleaceae

Parts used Fruit, oil, leaf

Actions Nutritious, demulcent, emollient, antiseptic, astringent, febrifuge, antioxidant, cholagogue, hypotensive, hypocholesterolaemic.

Digestion Soothes irritated and inflamed conditions such as indigestion, heartburn, gastritis, colitis and peptic ulcers. • Warm enemas help to relieve constipation. • Traditionally used as a gastric lavage for poisoning by alkalis/corrosives to soothe irritated mucosae and hasten elimination. • Stimulates bile flow; used for liver and gall bladder problems. Alternated with lemon juice to dissolve and encourage the passing of gallstones. • Leaves lower blood sugar; helpful in diabetes.

Circulation Cold-pressed oil is high in oleic acid; can lower harmful cholesterol, blood pressure and reduce risk of atherosclerosis, clots, heart attacks and strokes. • Leaves relax blood vessels and lower blood pressure; used for hypertension, angina and other circulatory problems. • Hot infusion of leaves increases sweating and reduces fevers.

Respiratory system Soothes harsh, dry coughs, laryngitis and croup. • Reduces catarrh.

Immune system Antioxidants make cell membranes less susceptible to destruction by free radicals. May reduce development of cancer and retard ageing.

Externally Applied to boils, eczema, cold sores, dry skin, brittle nails, insect bites and stings and minor burns to speed healing. • Warm oil dropped into the ear softens wax; used with essential oils such as garlic or lavender to relieve earache. • Massaged over kidneys for bed-wetting. • Infusion of leaves used as a mouthwash for bleeding/infected gums; and gargle for sore throats.

Origanum majorana

Sweet marjoram

With its white flowers and grey-green leaves Marjoram is a half-hardy annual in cool temperate areas and a perennial found growing wild in warmer areas of Europe and the USA. The ancient Greeks used it to nourish the brain and remedy the digestion.

Family Lamiaceae

Parts used Flower, leaf

Actions Digestive, carminative, tonic, stimulant, diaphoretic, antispasmodic, diuretic, antiviral, antioxidant, expectorant.

Digestion Antispasmodic and warming; used for indigestion, poor appetite, wind and colic, nausea, diarrhoea and constipation.

Circulation Stimulates blood flow and taken hot clears toxins via the skin; used for poor circulation, chilblains, arthritis and gout.

Mental and emotional Traditionally used to calm unwanted sexual desire and to ease loneliness, bereavement and heartbreak. • Relaxes mental and physical tension; relieves insomnia, restlessness, anxiety, depression, aching muscles and stress-related symptoms such as indigestion, colic, headaches, migraine, period pains, PMS, poor concentration and memory.

Immune system Antioxidants minimize damage from free radicals and retard ageing. • Enhances immunity and increases circulation. • Essential oils are antimicrobial against bacteria such as TB, viruses such as herpes simplex and fungal infections such as candida; protect against winter infections such as coughs and colds. • Clears phlegm, soothes coughs and relieves sinusitis and fevers. • Probiotic.

Urinary system Antiseptic diuretic for infections and fluid retention. Clears toxins via urine.

Externally Diluted essential oils can be massaged into painful joints, aching muscles, sprains and strains.

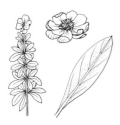
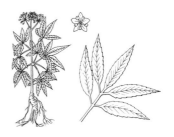

Paeonia lactiflora, officinalis
Peony

There are 33 species of Peony native to Europe, China and North America. *P. lactiflora*, with red, white or pink-scented flowers, was cultivated in China from 900 BCE.

Family Paeoniaceae

Parts used Root, seed, flower

Actions *P. officinalis*: diuretic, emmenagogue, bitter tonic, alterative, astringent; *P. lactiflora* cultivated root: liver tonic, astringent, antispasmodic, sedative, antiseptic, diuretic, nourishing; wild harvested root: anodyne, cooling, febrifuge;

Digestion Liver and gall bladder remedy; dissolves gallstones. • Root reduces pain and spasm in the stomach and intestines, use for diarrhoea, dysentery and stress-related gastric ulcers.

Circulation Improves venous return; benefits varicose veins and haemorrhoids. • Bai-shao used in Traditional Chinese Medicine for hypertension, hypertensive headaches, fevers, dizziness due to poor circulation and blood deficiency with liver heat.

Mental and emotional Bai-shao is calming; relaxes spasm in the chest, gut and uterus and has anticonvulsive properties. • Traditional remedy for spasms, epilepsy, nervous twitches and St Vitus's dance.

Immune system Root is anti-inflammatory, antibacterial and antiviral. Clears signs of heat such as boils. • Used for stiff joints.

Urinary system Diuretic; helps dissolve stones.

Reproductive system Stimulates uterine muscles; aids contractions in childbirth and expulsion of the placenta. • Bai-shao reduces painful periods and night sweats.

Externally A knife wound with bleeding and pain is commonly treated with bai-shao in Chinese Traditional Medicine.

CAUTION Avoid in early pregnancy.

Panax ginseng
Korean ginseng

For centuries in the East, top-grade Ginseng roots have been valued more highly than gold. There are many different grades of Ginseng – Wild ginseng being considered the best.

Family Araliaceae

Parts used Root

Actions Tonic, adaptogen, alterative, stimulant, immunostimulant, rejuvenative.

Digestion Reduces blood sugar; useful for diabetics. • Improves the appetite and digestion and lowers harmful cholesterol.

Mental and emotional Chinese 'qi' tonic. Adaptogen; increases energy and resilience to stress. • Optimizes pituitary and adrenal function when stressed. • Increases efficiency of nerve impulses, enhancing overall mental and physical performance, memory, stamina and muscular strength. • Excellent when undergoing harsh physical training, recovering from illness or surgery, studying for exams or taking on a large project at work. • Rejuvenating tonic; reduces the impact of the ageing process.

Respiratory system Acts as a tonic to the lungs, reducing wheezing and shortness of breath.

Immune system Immune enhancer. Some 3,000 scientific studies confirm its ability to increase resistance to stress caused by extremes of temperature, excessive exertion, illness, hunger, mental strain and emotional problems. • Increases white blood cell action. • Improves liver function, aiding resistance to hepatotoxins and radiation. • Reduces depression of bone marrow when on anticancer drugs. • Decreases allergic responses.

Reproductive system Saponins stimulate sexual function in men and women; increase sperm production. • Reduces menopausal symptoms such as depression.

CAUTION Avoid in acute inflammatory conditions such as bronchitis.

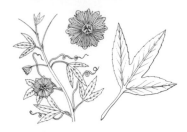
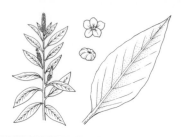

Passiflora incarnata
Passion flower

This perennial climber indigenous to South America has stunningly beautiful, intricate flowers. It derives its name from the resemblance of the centre of the flower to the cross and crown of thorns, symbolizing the Passion of Christ. This prompted its Spanish discoverers in Peru to send it to Pope Paul V in 1605.

Family Passifloraceae

Parts used Vine, flower

Actions Anodyne, anticonvulsive, sedative, antispasmodic, anxiolytic, hypotensive.

Digestion For stress-related digestive problems including wind, colic and indigestion.

Circulation Relaxes tension through the arterial system; reduces blood pressure and nervous palpitations.

Mental and emotional An excellent relaxant and sedative for stress-related and painful conditions.
• Improves circulation and nutrition to the nerves.
• Calms nervous anxiety, restlessness and agitation.
• Improves concentration and combats exam nerves.
• Soothes pain in headaches, neuralgia, shingles, muscular aches, backache and period pains. • Cooling in conditions of excess heat, inflammation, anger, intolerance and irritability. • Non-addictive tranquillizer for chronic insomnia. For best results, take during the day as well as before retiring. • Antispasmodic for Parkinson's disease, muscle twitching and cramps, high blood pressure and colic.

Respiratory system Antispasmodic; relieves irritating and nervous coughs, croup and asthma.

Drug interactions Avoid with monoamine oxidase-inhibiting antidepressants.

Phytolacca decandra
Poke root

This striking herb, native to North America, has reddish-purple berries, which are poisonous when raw. It is a potent remedy for the immune system and is being researched for its potential in treating cancer, HIV, bilharzia and arthritis.

Family Phytolaccaceae

Parts used Root

Actions Alterative, anodyne, anti-inflammatory, antirheumatic, antitumour, antiviral, laxative, expectorant, hypnotic, immunostimulant, lymphatic decongestant, narcotic, purgative, spermicide.

Respiratory system Strengthens immunity and combats acute and chronic infections; used for sore throats, throat infections, colds and flu viruses.

Musculoskeletal system Phytolaccosides have potent anti-inflammatory action. Detoxifying and anti-inflammatory for rheumatic and arthritic conditions.

Immune system Immune enhancing and cleansing. Supports the lymphatic system in its detoxifying and immune work. Used in swollen lymph nodes, tonsillitis, mumps, swollen breast and mastitis. • The proteins are antiviral; they can inhibit the replication of the influenza and herpes simplex viruses and poliovirus.
• Used in HIV and cancers including leukaemia and liver cancer. • The peptide PAFP-s has antifungal activity.

Externally Antifungal, antiseptic and anti-inflammatory wash used for athlete's foot, spots, acne, boils, abscesses, psoriasis, eczema, herpes, shingles, chickenpox, measles, tumours, impetigo and scabies, swelling sprains and strains.

CAUTION Only use in small doses. Avoid internal use during pregnancy, lactation and gastrointestinal irritation. Do not apply to broken skin.

Drug interactions Do not use with immunosuppressive drugs.

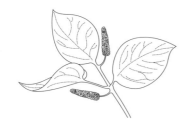

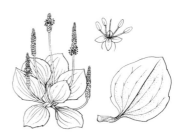

Piper longum
Long pepper

Native to tropical India, this has warming and energizing properties. It acts as a stimulant and a tonic for those feeling cold and run-down.

Family Piperaceae

Parts used Root, seed

Actions Stimulant, carminative, laxative, diuretic, febrifuge, tonic, expectorant, anthelmintic, digestive, antiseptic, emmenagogue, rejuvenative, analgesic, cardiac stimulant, hypocholesterolaemic.

Digestion Enhances appetite, digestion and absorption up to 30 per cent. Piperine stimulates an enzyme that enhances the uptake of amino acids from the gastrointestinal tract. Used for anorexia, dyspepsia, flatulence, constipation, colic and weak digestion. • Antimicrobial for amoebae, worms and candida. • Hepatoprotective, enhancing the liver's ability to break down toxins; reduces liver damage.

Circulation Vasodilatory. • Stimulates circulation and reduces harmful cholesterol. • Used for anaemia.

Mental and emotional Promotes energy and vitality. • Reduces tension, anxiety and insomnia.

Respiratory system Decongestant for colds, catarrh, bronchial congestion and bronchitis. • Traditionally used in milk to reduce bronchospasm in asthma.

Immune system Anti-inflammatory for gout, arthritis and muscle and back pain. • Enhances immunity; activates macrophages and phagocytosis. • Found to be helpful in the treatment of hepatitis. • Broad spectrum antibiotic activity against gram+ and gram- bacteria, including Staphylococcus aureus. • Reduces allergic conditions including hay fever and eczema. • Antioxidant and rejuvenative. • Reduces fevers; traditionally used for typhoid and chronic fevers.

Reproductive system May have a contraceptive effect; reduces sperm count. • Reputed to be an aphrodisiac. • Antispasmodic for dysmenorrhoea.

CAUTION May increase drug absorption. Use cautiously in acidity. Avoid in pregnancy and lactation.

Plantago major
Greater plantain

This common perennial with cylindrical spikes of seeds grows in lawns and on cultivated and waste ground. It is historically famous as a wound healer and an antidote to poisons.

Family Plantaginaceae

Parts used Leaf, seed of P. psyllium

Actions Leaf: astringent, alterative, diuretic, demulcent, refrigerant, detoxifying, decongestant, expectorant, antiseptic, antispasmodic. Seed: bulk laxative, demulient.

Digestion Leaf: astringent and soothing. Counters irritation and inflammation in the stomach and bowels; used for gastritis, diarrhoea, colitis and stomach and bowel infections. • Reduces spasm and colic. • Seeds are used as a bulk laxative.

Respiratory system Leaf depresses mucous secretion in colds, catarrh, sinusitis, bronchial congestion and allergies such as hay fever and asthma. Helps prevent glue ear and ear infections. • Mucilage protects mucosae from irritation; soothes cough reflex. • Expectorant and antispasmodic for coughs and asthma. • Antiseptic for colds, tonsillitis and chest infections.

Immune system Leaf: polysaccharides have an immunomodulating effect. • Tannins reduce swelling and inflammation, staunch bleeding and promote healing. • Clears heat and toxins; reduces fevers, infections and skin problems. • Antiviral against herpes viruses and adenoviruses, and urinary tract infections.

Reproductive system Astringent for excessive menstrual bleeding. • Useful for prostatitis enlargement.

Externally Used for cuts, stings and insect bites.

CAUTION Take seeds with plenty of fluid to prevent bowel obstruction.

Drug interactions Care needed with patients on insulin, as seeds can lower blood sugar. Separate by 2 hours from other drugs. May inhibit absorption.

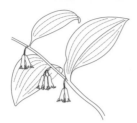

Polygonum multiflorum
Polygonum

A perennial vine, native to Japan, Vietnam and China, this is highly valued as an adaptogen.

Family Polygonaceae

Parts used Processed root

Actions Adaptogen, immune tonic, rejuvenative, hypocholesterolaemic, bitter, alterative, antibacterial, antioxidant, aphrodisiac, demulcent, cholagogue, laxative, astringent, blood tonic, hypoglycaemic, kidney tonic, sedative.

Digestion Protects liver against damage from toxins, chemicals, alcohol and drugs. • Enhances liver and gall bladder function. • Reduces gut irritation. • Useful in constipation from dryness. • Lowers blood sugar.

Circulation Reduces blood pressure and harmful cholesterol; prevents atherosclerosis. • Increases cerebral circulation; used for dizziness with tinnitus and anaemia.

Mental and emotional Increases energy and resilience to stress. • Used for nervous exhaustion and insomnia. Excellent tonic for the elderly and during convalescence. • Improves memory.

Musculoskeletal system Strengthens bones, muscles and tendons.

Immune system Adaptogenic and antioxidant; enhances immunity and protects against cancer. • Antiageing through the inhibition of brain monoamine oxidase. • Increases secretion of adrenal and thyroid hormones; enhances T lymphocyte and macrophage activity.

Reproductive system Strengthening tonic and aphrodisiac for impotence, low sperm count, infertility and menopausal problems. • For signs of kidney weakness including low libido, poor vision, weak knees and grey hair.

CAUTION May cause diarrhoea.

Drug interactions Avoid with tetracycline, statins and acetaminophen.

Prunella vulgaris
Selfheal

A small perennial, with purple flowers, growing wild in Europe, North America and China.

Family Lamiaceae

Parts used Aerial parts

Actions Astringent, tonic, anti-inflammatory, relaxant, antibiotic, diuretic, digestive, liver tonic, antiallergenic, antioxidant, restorative.

Digestion Astringent for diarrhoea and inflammatory bowel problems such as colitis. • Bitters stimulate the liver and gall bladder.

Mental and emotional Used for headaches, particularly when related to tension, vertigo, oversensitivity to light and high blood pressure. • Used in China for hyperactivity in children.

Immune system Enhances immunity. Research indicates a potent antiviral action, including activity against HIV, and the polysaccharides have an immunomodulatory effect. • Rosmarinic acid contributes to its antioxidant effects. • Research indicates antimutagenic effects, indicating possible anticancer use. • Recommended in lowered immunity, HIV, chronic fatigue syndrome and allergies. • Effective antibiotic against a range of bacteria. • Used for swollen glands, mumps, glandular fever and mastitis. • Detoxifying; clears inflammatory skin problems. • Reduces fevers.

Urinary system Urosolic acid is a diuretic that has anticancer properties; clears toxins and excess uric acid via the kidneys. Recommended for gout.

Reproductive system Astringent; curbs heavy menstrual bleeding.

Externally Traditional wound remedy. • Gargle used for sore throats; mouthwash for mouth ulcers and bleeding gums. • Tea/fresh plant used to stop bleeding, reduce swelling from minor injuries, burns, bites and stings, piles, varicose veins and ulcers. • Drops used for inflammatory eye problems such as conjunctivitis.

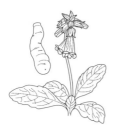

Rehmannia

Rehmannia glutinosa

Native to China, where it is famous as a yin and blood tonic, increasing energy and immunity, and a strengthening tonic for children.

Family Scrophulariaceae

Parts used Root; uncured or cured

Actions Haemostatic, antioxidant, antibacterial, hepatoprotective, immune tonic, antipyretic, demulcent, alterative, laxative, anti-inflammatory.

Digestion Astringent for diarrhoea. • Increases appetite. • Regulates blood sugar.

Circulation Improves coronary blood flow; helps prevent cardiovascular disease.

Respiratory system Strengthens lung energy; prevents colds, flu, fevers, coughs, bronchitis, pneumonia, asthma and TB. • Reduces phlegm.

Musculoskeletal system Strengthens bones, muscles and tendons; prevents muscle weakness and prolapse.

Immune system Protects against infections such as glandular fever and post-viral fatigue. • Inhibits formation of tumours and prevents immunosuppression by chemotherapy. • Used for inflammatory conditions associated with depletion. • Uncured root useful in autoimmune disease such as rheumatoid arthritis, and allergies. • Protects and supports the liver and adrenal glands.

Urinary system Strengthens kidneys, stems bleeding and reduces urinary frequency and incontinence.

Reproductive system Prepared root used in Chinese Medicine for low kidney energy and yin deficiency, night sweats, vertigo, tinnitus, lower back pain; regulates menstrual flow. • Curbs bleeding in heavy periods. • Reduces menopausal hot flushes.

CAUTION Best prepared with Cardamom or Ginger to prevent indigestion.

Drug interactions Use cautiously with immunosuppressant drugs.

Rhodiola

Rhodiola rosea

A perennial plant with red, pink or yellowish flowers, native to the Himalayas and found growing at high elevations in Asia, Europe and North America. It has long been considered a tonic to increase physical and mental endurance and strength.

Family Crassulaceae

Parts used Root, stem, leaf, flower, seed

Actions Adaptogen, tonic, antioxidant, antitumour, brain tonic, thymoleptic, immunostimulant.

Circulation Cardioprotective; normalizes heart rate after intense exercise. • Protects against altitude sickness. • Used in anaemia and cardiovascular disorder. • Combats the effects of excess adrenaline, which causes raised blood pressure and blood lipids.

Mental and emotional Reputed to be more powerful than other adaptogens. Increases ability to deal with stress. • Increases blood supply to the brain and muscles. • Improves memory and concentration and increases attention span. • Recommended for elevating mood in depression. • Useful sedative for insomnia in higher doses.

Musculoskeletal system Energy tonic; increases protein synthesis, useful in increasing strength and endurance in athletes and the elderly. Recommended for combating fatigue, physical stress, chronic fatigue syndrome and fibromyalgia.

Immune system Stimulates immunity directly by increasing natural killer cells, improving T-cell immunity and increasing resilience to stress. • Helps combat infections, including TB. • Helps prevent cancer as it has antitumour, antimetastatic and antimutagenic properties, which increase resistance to toxins and chemicals that could be potentially harmful. • Supportive during chemotherapy or radiotherapy; shortens recovery time of suppressed white blood cells following chemotherapy or radiation therapy.

CAUTION Do not take simultaneously with mineral supplements.

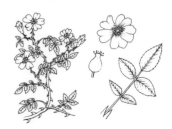
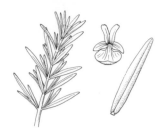

Rosa spp.
Rose

Roses have long been valued for their cooling properties, for strengthening the heart and refreshing the spirit.

Family Rosaceae

Parts used Hip, leaf, flower

Actions Diaphoretic, carminative, stimulant, emmenagogue, laxative, decongestant, febrifuge, anti-inflammatory, astringent, antimicrobial, thymoleptic, analgesic.

Digestion Combats infection and helps re-establish normal gut flora. • Tannins reduce hyperacidity and stomach overactivity causing excessive hunger and mouth ulcers. Useful for diarrhoea and enteritis. • Rose hip syrup or decoction of empty seed cases relieves diarrhoea, stomach cramps, constipation and nausea.

Mental and emotional Used for insomnia, depression, irritability, anger and mental and physical fatigue.

Respiratory system Stimulates action of the mucociliary escalator, antimicrobial and decongestant; helps to prevent and relieve colds, flu, sore throats, catarrh, coughs and bronchitis.

Immune system Combats infection and clears heat and toxins. Hips are famous for an immune-enhancing syrup; a rich source of vitamin C, A, B and K. • Hips have anti-inflammatory effects; reduce pain and increase flexibility in osteoarthritis.

Urinary system Flowers and seeds relieve infections and fluid retention; hasten the elimination of toxins. • Reduces inflammation and dissolves stones.

Reproductive system Flowers relieve uterine congestion that causes pain, heavy and irregular periods. • Antispasmodic and relaxing for menstrual cramps and PMS. • Cooling for menopausal hot flushes, night sweats and mood swings.

Externally Rosewater cleanses and tones skin; clears infection and inflammation in acne, spots, boils, and sore eyes, minor cuts and wounds. • Reduces swelling of bruises and sprains.

Rosmarinus officinalis
Rosemary

Native to the Mediterranean, this perennial shrub has been recognized as a rejuvenating brain tonic since the ancient Egyptians.

Family Lamiaceae

Parts used Aerial parts

Actions Carminative, emmenagogue, antioxidant, cholagogue, decongestant, antispasmodic, antimicrobial, circulatory stimulant, febrifuge.

Digestion Tannins protect the gut lining from irritation and inflammation, reducing bleeding and diarrhoea. • Antimicrobial for infections. • Stimulates appetite, digestion and absorption, relieves flatulence and distension. • Enhances elimination. • Bitters stimulate bile flow from the liver and gall bladder, aid digestion of fats and clear toxins.

Circulation Stimulates blood flow to the head, reduces inflammation and muscle tension. Specific for migraines and headaches. • Stimulates general circulation, improving peripheral blood flow. • Used for varicose veins, chilblains and arteriosclerosis.

Mental and emotional Excellent brain tonic, improves concentration and memory. • Calms anxiety and lifts depression, relieves exhaustion and insomnia.

Respiratory system Volatile oils dispel infection. • Hot tea used for fevers, catarrh, sore throats, colds, flu and chest infections. • Helpful in asthma.

Immune system Volatile oils are antibacterial, antifungal and antiviral, and enhance immunity. • Antioxidant; may have potential as an anticancer remedy. Stimulates liver enzymes that detoxify poisons including carcinogens. • Relieves arthritis and gout.

Urinary system Enhances elimination of wastes.

Reproductive system Reduces heavy menstrual bleeding and relieves dysmenorrhoea.

Externally Diluted essential oil is rubbed onto the skin for joint pain, headaches and poor concentration.

CAUTION Avoid in pregnancy.

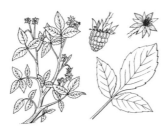
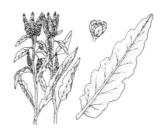

Rubus idaeus
Raspberry

Native to Europe and temperate Asia, Raspberry is well known for its delicious fruit, while the leaves have traditionally been valued for their astringent properties. They were given to relieve diarrhoea and were best known as a parturient, to prepare women for childbirth.

Family Rosaceae

Parts used Leaf, fruit

Actions Anti-inflammatory, astringent, birthing aid, decongestant, antiemetic, ophthalmic, antioxidant, antiseptic, antidiarrhoeal, diaphoretic, diuretic, choleretic, partus praeparator, hypoglycaemic.

Digestion Astringent. Protects gut lining from irritation and inflammation; relieves nausea and diarrhoea. • Helps normalize blood sugar levels. Manganese may effect glucose regulation.

Respiratory system Antiseptic astringent. Taken in hot tea for sore throats, colds, flu and catarrh.

Reproductive system Uterine astringent used for frequent or excessive menstruation, painful periods and other menstrual disorders. • Relieves nausea in pregnancy and helps prevent miscarriage. • Infusion of leaves in last 3 months of pregnancy tones uterine and pelvic muscles to prepare for childbirth. By relaxing over-tense muscles and toning over-relaxed muscles, the leaves enable the uterus to contract effectively during childbirth, easing and speeding the birth. • Taken afterwards, they stimulate the flow of breast milk and speed healing. • Raspberries are nutritious; useful in pregnancy to combat anaemia.

Externally Used as a gargle and mouthwash for sore throats, tonsillitis, mouth ulcers and inflamed gums. • Poultice/lotion used for sores, conjunctivitis, minor cuts and wounds, burns and varicose ulcers.

Rumex crispus
Yellow dock

A common inhabitant of hedgerows, meadows, ditches and roadsides in temperate areas. The leaves are well known for relieving nettle stings, while the whole plant has been valued since the ancient Greeks, for cleansing toxins and aiding digestion.

Family Polygonaceae

Parts used Root

Actions Alterative, antiscorbutic, astringent, antitumour, cholagogue, depurative, laxative, tonic.

Digestion Famous for its detoxifying properties. Gentle laxative properties due to anthraquinones, which stimulate peristalsis and cleanse the bowel. • Astringent tannins check irritation and inflammation, and curb diarrhoea. • Bitters stimulate the liver and benefit digestion. Used for liver and gall bladder complaints, headaches and lethargy.

Circulation Affinity with blood, enriching it with iron and clearing impurities. Traditionally used for anaemia, bleeding of the lungs and bleeding haemorrhoids. • Stimulates lymphatic circulation; reduces chronic lymphatic congestion and glandular swellings.

Immune system Invigorating tonic; cleansing and nutritive. • Traditionally used as an anticancer remedy. • Anti-inflammatory; useful in arthritis.

Urinary system Diuretic properties increase the elimination of toxins via the kidneys; useful for fluid retention, cystitis, gout and arthritis.

Skin Cleansing and anti-inflammatory as it aids elimination of toxins through the bowels and kidneys. For chronic skin diseases such as acne, eczema and psoriasis.

Externally Lotion used for swellings, skin rashes, cuts, sores, ulcers and infections. • Crushed leaves are applied to burns, scalds and nettle stings.

CAUTION Excess doses can cause gastric disturbance, nausea and dermatitis.

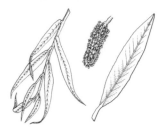
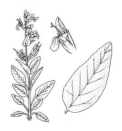

Salix alba and S. nigra
White and Black willow

White willow is a large, elegant tree that grows by riverbanks and in damp places throughout Europe, North Africa and Central Asia, while Black willow is native to eastern North America.

Family Salicaceae

Parts used Bark

Actions Febrifuge, analgesic, anti-inflammatory, astringent, tonic, stomachic, diuretic, anodyne, antiseptic, sedative.

Digestion Astringent tannins protect the gut lining from irritation and inflammation. Relieves diarrhoea and dysentery and stems bleeding.

Respiratory system Decongestant for head colds, flu and fevers. • Tonic to restore strength after illness.

Musculoskeletal system Pain reliever and anti-inflammatory for rheumatism, arthritis, gout, aching muscles, inflammatory stages of autoimmune diseases, backache, tendonitis, bursitis and sprains.

Immune system The original source of salicylic acid; used like aspirin for fevers, muscular aches and pains accompanying flu, headaches, inflammation and arthritic pain without side effects. • Traditionally used for intermittent fevers as in malaria.

Urinary system Diuretic; reduces fluid retention and helps to eliminate toxins from the body via the urinary system.

Externally Lotion used for cuts and wounds; gargles for sore throats; mouthwashes for mouth ulcers and bleeding gums; and poultices for inflamed joints.

CAUTION Avoid in bleeding problems and if allergic to salicylates. Children and teenagers with chickenpox, flu or any undiagnosed illness should not take it without first consulting a practitioner due to theoretical risk of Reye's syndrome.

Drug interactions Use with caution with non-steroidal anti-inflammatory drugs such as ibuprofen or naproxen.

Salvia officinalis
Sage

An evergreen perennial shrub, native to southern Europe and the Mediterranean. It was regarded as the 'immortality herb' by the ancient Greeks.

Family Lamiaceae

Parts used Leaves

Actions Antimicrobial, astringent, antiseptic, bitter tonic, digestive, antioxidant, rejuvenative, diuretic, phytoestrogenic, antihydrotic, carminative, cholagogue, vasodilator.

Digestion Improves appetite, digestion and absorption. • Relaxes tension and colic. • Relieves bloating and wind. • Beneficial effect on the liver and pancreatic function. Lowers blood sugar.

Mental and emotional Reduces anxiety, lifts depression and decreases excessive salivation.

Respiratory system Decongestant, antimicrobial and expectorant; excellent for catarrh, colds and chest infections.

Immune system Antibacterial, antiviral and antifungal for colds, flu, fevers, sore throats and chest infections. Effective against candida, herpes simplex type 2 and influenza virus II. • Antioxidant actions explain its rejuvenative effects.

Urinary system Aids elimination of toxins via the kidneys; useful for arthritis and gout.

Reproductive system Hormone balancing and antispasmodic for irregular, scanty and painful periods. • Used for menopausal problems such as night sweats and insomnia. • Reduces excessive lactation.

Externally Antiseptic lotion for cuts, burns, insect bites, skin problems, ulcers and sunburn; gargle for sore throats; mouthwash for inflamed gums and ulcers. • Poultice used for sprains, swellings and ulcers.

CAUTION May be toxic in large dosages or over a prolonged period. Avoid in pregnancy and breast-feeding and with epilepsy.

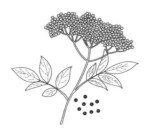

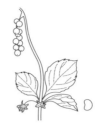

Sambucus nigra
Elder

The Elder with its abundance of white flowers has been called the 'medicine chest of the country people', as it has many health benefits.

Family Caprifoliaceae

Parts used Flower, berry

Actions Relaxant, antioxidant, adaptogen, decongestant, diuretic, immune enhancing, alterative, astringent, anti-inflammatory, antimicrobial, febrifuge.

Digestion Flowers are antispasmodic and astringent to the gut, protecting it against irritation and inflammation; useful for heartburn, indigestion, gastritis, diarrhoea, gastroenteritis, colic and wind.

Circulation Anthocyanins in berries protect blood vessel walls against oxidative stress, preventing vascular disease. • Berries reduce harmful cholesterol and help prevent atherosclerosis.

Mental and emotional Flowers are calming and soothing for tension, anxiety and depression. • Induces sleep. • Berries increase resilience to stress.

Respiratory system Hot infusion of flowers is beneficial at the onset of colds, fevers, flu, tonsillitis and laryngitis. • Decongestant and relaxant effects relieve catarrh, bronchial congestion and asthma.

Immune system Flowers and berries are antimicrobial and decongestant. • Berries activate immunity by increasing cytokine production and prevent damage caused by free radicals. Their proteins help regulate the immune response. • Berries have antiviral action, inhibiting colds and influenza A and B and herpes virus; may be helpful in HIV.

Urinary system Flowers enhance kidney function, relieve fluid retention and eliminate toxins and heat.

Externally Used as a gargle for sore throats; mouthwash for mouth ulcers and inflamed gums; eyewash for conjunctivitis and sore, tired eyes.

CAUTION Leaves may cause a reaction in sensitive skins. Avoid use of the root and bark.

Schisandra chinensis
Schisandra

Native to China, the red berries with their five tastes are considered to balance all bodily systems in Traditional Chinese Medicine.

Family Schisandraceae

Parts used Fruit, seed

Actions Adaptogen, antibacterial, antidepressant, antitussive, aphrodisiac, antioxidant, anti-inflammatory, astringent, antiasthmatic, hepatotonic, immune tonic, rejuvenative, hypoglycaemic, sedative.

Digestion Lignans in the seeds have liver-protective properties against chemical toxins. • Besides hepatitis and other liver ailments, Schisandra is also helpful in intestinal infections including chronic gastritis.

Circulation Reduces nervous palpitations, improves blood flow through coronary arteries and protects the heart from ischaemic damage.

Mental and emotional Increases energy, endurance and resilience to stress. • Prevents altitude sickness. • Used for depletion from stress, chronic fatigue syndrome, anxiety, depression, irritability, dizziness and Ménière's disease. • Anticonvulsive; may help in Parkinson's disease. • Improves memory and concentration. • Helpful in neuralgia, insomnia and nervous palpitations.

Respiratory system Boosts immunity, reduces allergies and moistens lungs; used in chronic coughs and allergic asthma.

Immune system Prevents damage from free radicals. • Improves liver regeneration and recovery after hepatitis. Enhances glutathione protection in the liver, stimulates glycogen and protein synthesis and may protect against liver cancer. • Stimulates production of interferon and lymphocytes. • Anti-inflammatory.

Reproductive system Relieves night sweats, frequent urination, low libido, spermatorrhoea, premature ejaculation and low sperm count. • Enhances fertility.

CAUTION Avoid in pregnancy and epilepsy.

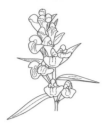

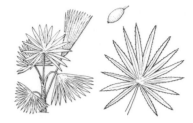

Scutellaria baicalensis
Baikal skullcap

A small perennial, native to Siberia, Russia, North China, Mongolia and Japan, it is used in Traditional Chinese and Tibetan medicine to clear 'damp heat', and as a strengthening nerve and immune tonic.

Family Lamiaceae

Parts used Root

Actions Antihistamine, antioxidant, anti-inflammatory, sedative, antitumour, anticlotting agent, vasodilator, antibacterial, diuretic, febrifuge, choleretic.

Digestion Clears heat from the gut in bowel infections, diarrhoea and dysentery, and is indicated in chronic hepatitis and other liver problems.

Urinary system Antiseptic diuretic for urinary tract infections, dysuria and haematuria.

Circulation Protective effect on the heart and circulation. Dilates peripheral arteries, reduces blood pressure and prevents clots.

Mental and emotional Energizing nerve tonic and sedative for depletion from stress, anxiety, convulsions, cramps and nervous heart conditions.

Immune system Antihistamine for allergies including eczema, asthma, hay fever, urticaria and rhinitis. Inhibits release of histamine from mast cells. • Useful for autoimmune problems such as rheumatoid arthritis and lupus. • Antibacterial against a wide range of infecting organisms including Staphylococcus aureus, Pseudomonas aeruginosa and Streptococcus pneumoniae. Has an affinity with the respiratory, urinary and digestive tracts. • Reduces fevers.

Reproductive system Traditionally used to prevent miscarriage.

Eyes Clears soreness and inflammation associated with 'liver heat'.

Serenoa repens
Saw palmetto

A small plant bearing dark blue-black berries native to North America. Its benefits were first discovered by farmers who observed that animals that fed on the berries looked healthy despite the summer drought.

Family Arecaceae

Parts used Berry

Actions Anti-inflammatory, adaptogen, rejuvenative, anabolic, antiandrogenic, decongestant, diuretic, nutritive, digestive, demulcent, antitumour, antibacterial, immunostimulant, aphrodisiac.

Digestion Enhances appetite and digestion. Used for anorexia, diarrhoea and gall bladder problems.

Mental and emotional Reduces tension; increases resilience to stress and induces sleep.

Respiratory system Soothes irritation and resolves infection. • Expectorant, clears catarrh. • Used in whooping cough, laryngitis, chronic coughs, TB, bronchitis and asthma.

Immune system A tonic to increase strength and weight. • Adaptogenic; enhances immunity and endurance. Used for frequent infections and allergies.

Urinary system Soothing diuretic; relieves cystitis, irritable bladder, infections and incontinence. • Clears toxins and helps resolve skin problems.

Reproductive system Tonic for low libido, low sperm count and erectile dysfunction. • Inhibits prolactin; may suppress milk flow in nursing mothers. • Specific for benign prostatic hypertrophy; improves the flow of urine, relieves pain, reduces swelling and inhibits further growth of the prostate by increasing breakdown of dihydrotestosterone (DHT) without affecting prostate-specific antigen (PSA) readings. Reduces inflammation in prostatitis, orchitis and epididymitis. • Used with Vitex for polycystic ovaries, hirsutism, acne and in fertility problems related to excess androgens.

CAUTION Avoid when breast-feeding.

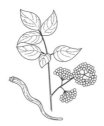
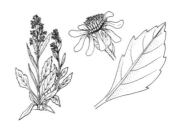

Smilax ornata
Sarsaparilla

A climbing vine native to South and Central America, the Caribbean and parts of Asia.

Family Smilacaceae

Parts used Rhizome

Actions Alterative, antimicrobial, anti-inflammatory, antiseptic, antitumour, astringent, carminative, cholagogue, demulcent, diaphoretic, diuretic, rejuvenative, stimulant, digestive, tonic, antirheumatic.

Digestion Supports and protects the liver. • Reduces oxidative load in the bowel. • Nutritive; increases the body's metabolic processes.

Mental and emotional Strengthening tonic for debility and depression, especially in menopause.

Musculoskeletal system Increases muscle mass and improves strength and athletic performance. • Diuretic properties help clear excess uric acid helpful in gout and arthritis.

Immune system Antimicrobial, anti-inflammatory and detoxifying. • Steroidal saponins bind to toxins in the gut and inhibit their absorption. Beneficial in autoimmune problems such as psoriasis, rheumatoid arthritis and ulcerative colitis, which can be associated with toxicity. • Saponins have antibiotic activity.

Urinary system Diuretic; clears toxins via the kidneys. Recommended for infections, stones, renal colic, bed-wetting and urinary incontinence.

Reproductive system Tonic and aphrodisiac for low libido, impotence and erectile dysfunction. • Regulates menstrual cycle. Used for menorrhagia, menstrual cramps, ovarian cysts, pelvic inflammatory disease, PMS and infertility. • Helpful during menopause for hot flushes and night sweats.

Skin Anti-inflammatory and detoxifying. Useful in eczema and psoriasis; relieves itching and dryness.

CAUTION Avoid during pregnancy.

Drug interactions Avoid with warfarin.

Solidago virgaurea
Goldenrod

A perennial with bright yellow flowers native to North America. It was traditionally used to stop bleeding and heal wounds.

Family Asteraceae

Parts used Aerial parts

Actions Analgesic, anthelmintic, anticatarrhal, antifungal, anti-inflammatory, antioxidant, antiseptic, astringent, carminative, decongestant, diaphoretic, diuretic, expectorant, alterative, stimulant.

Digestion Useful for maintaining gut flora and treating candida, colic, indigestion, diarrhoea, gastroenteritis, nausea, peptic ulcers and worms.
• Stimulates bile flow from the liver.

Circulation Reduces blood pressure.

Respiratory system Decongestant, expectorant and antimicrobial; helps combat infection in throat infections, colds, flu, catarrh, sinusitis, middle ear infections, catarrhal deafness, hay fever, coughs and bronchitis. Also used in asthma.

Immune system Astringent and antimicrobial; combats infection in the digestive, respiratory and urinary tracts. • Anti-inflammatory and analgesic; can be helpful in rheumatoid and osteoarthritis.

Urinary system Antiseptic diuretic; aids elimination of toxins; useful in gout, inflammatory problems, cystitis, acute and chronic urinary tract infections, bed-wetting, bladder weakness and incontinence. • Helps dissolve kidney and bladder stones.

Reproductive system Used for benign prostate enlargement. • Regulates the menstrual cycle, relieves menstrual cramps and heavy and irregular periods.

Externally Poultice/compress/lotion used for arthritis, boils, burns, fungal infections, eczema, swellings and wounds. • Gargle used for sore throat, laryngitis and candida; and mouthwash for toothache.

CAUTION Avoid in oedema from heart or kidney failure and in known allergy.

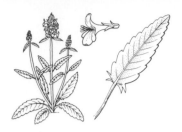

Stachys betonica
Wood betony

Native to Europe, Wood betony grows wild in hedgerows and meadows and is a specific for headaches.

Family Lamiaceae

Parts used Aerial parts

Actions Digestive, circulatory stimulant, nerve tonic, sedative, astringent, liver tonic, anthelmintic, antiseptic, carminative, cholagogue, diuretic, emmenagogue, expectorant.

Digestion Enhances appetite and digestion. • Astringent tannins protect the gut lining from inflammation and infection. • Used for indigestion, colic, wind, heartburn, diarrhoea and parasites. • Reduces liver and gall bladder problems.

Mental and emotional Tonic and sedative to nerves. Relieves pain, particularly in trigeminal neuralgia and sciatica. • Reduces tension and anxiety; lifts depression. • Improves circulation to the head, stimulates liver function and reduces tension; specific for headaches whether from poor circulation, a sluggish liver or tension. • Improves memory and concentration.

Respiratory system Astringent and antiseptic. • In hot tea it stimulates the circulation and helps throw off colds, catarrh, sinusitis and coughs.

Urinary system Diuretic; aids elimination of toxins and excess uric acid, helpful in gout and arthritis.

Reproductive system Relieves period pain and PMS. • Stimulates uterine muscle, brings on delayed periods. • Relaxing for menopausal flushes, insomnia and depression.

Externally Stems bleeding, speeds repair and inhibits infection of cuts and wounds, ulcers, varicose veins and haemorrhoids. • Lotions/creams used for bruises, sprains and strains. • Draws splinters and thorns. • Traditionally taken as snuff for nosebleeds and headaches.

CAUTION Avoid during pregnancy.

Stellaria media
Chickweed

Native to Eurasia, Chickweed is highly nutritious and considered a delicacy in Europe. It is thought to improve eyesight, as it is rich in vitamin A.

Family Caryophyllaceae

Parts used Aerial parts

Actions Demulcent, refrigerant, anti-inflammatory, diuretic, astringent, carminative, depurative, emmenagogue, expectorant, laxative, ophthalmic.

Digestion Soothing aid to digestion and laxative. Relieves wind, constipation, inflammatory problems such as gastritis, colitis, acid indigestion, irritable bowel syndrome. Clears excess heat in the liver and gall bladder.

Respiratory system Expectorant and soothing; helpful in sore throats, laryngitis, bronchitis, asthma, harsh dry coughs and pleurisy. • Reduces fevers and thirst.

Urinary system Soothing diuretic; relieves fluid retention, cystitis and irritable bladder. • Aids the elimination of toxins via the kidneys, which helps skin problems and arthritis. • Traditional remedy for obesity.

Reproductive system Traditionally a post-partum blood purifier. • Promotes milk flow in nursing mothers.

Skin Excellent cooling remedy for inflammatory skin conditions such as eczema, heat rashes, urticaria, sunburn, boils and spots.

Externally A specific for itchy skin conditions including eczema, roseola, fragile superficial veins, burns, scalds, ulcers, piles and abscesses. • Healing for wounds, and ulcers. • Expressed juice is used as an eyewash for inflammatory eye problems. • Poultice and strong infusions added to baths reduce inflammation and encourage tissue repair. • Helps bring poisons and pus to the surface.

CAUTION Excess doses can cause diarrhoea and vomiting. Avoid in pregnancy and breast-feeding.

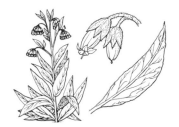

Symphytum officinale
Comfrey

Comfrey is native to Europe and western Asia, growing wild in damp meadows and by streams. It is highly valued for its ability to promote the repair of wounds, ulcers and broken bones.

Family Boraginaceae

Parts used Root (external use only), leaf

Actions Demulcent, emollient, haemostatic, nutritive, refrigerant, expectorant, astringent, pectoral tonic, alterative, anti-inflammatory.

Digestion Mucilage soothes irritation and inflammation. • Astringent tannins stop bleeding and protect surfaces against inflammation and infection. • Cooling and soothing remedy for heartburn, gastritis, peptic ulcers, diarrhoea and ulcerative colitis. • Rich in nutrients, nourishing and restorative.

Respiratory system Mucilage soothes irritation; relieves sore throats, laryngitis, tonsillitis, pleurisy, harsh, irritating coughs, bronchitis, whooping cough and asthma. • Rosmarinic acid decreases microvascular pulmonary injury.

Musculoskeletal system Allantoin is a remarkable cell proliferant; stimulates the production of cells responsible for forming collagen and connective tissue, cartilage and bone and speeds repair in injury. Excellent for broken or fractured bones. • Rosmarinic acid decreases inflammation. Reduces pain and swelling in arthritis, gout, carpal tunnel syndrome, tendonitis, sprains and strains.

Urinary system Soothes mucous membranes; relieves cystitis and irritable bladder.

Externally Promotes wound healing and tissue regeneration. Prime first-aid remedy for healing cuts, wounds, bruises, burns, scalds, sunburn and ulcers, with minimal scar formation. Soothing and rejuvenating to dry, sore, scarred and wrinkled skin.

CAUTION Avoid root for internal use. Avoid use on broken skin and during pregnancy.

Tabebuia impetiginosa
Pau d'arco

An evergreen flowering tree native to Brazil and Argentina, used as an immune enhancer, for fighting infection and preventing cancer.

Family Bignoniaceae

Parts used Inner bark

Actions Immune enhancing, antitumour, antioxidant, antimicrobial, antiparasitic, laxative, antimalarial, antischistosomal, anti-inflammatory, anticoagulant.

Digestion Antimicrobial for infections associated with diarrhoea, dysentery and peptic ulcers. Combats intestinal parasites and candida. • Reduces blood sugar; indicated in diabetes. • Reduces inflammation; useful in gastritis, ulcers, acidity, enteritis. • Laxative.

Circulation Increases oxygen supply to the body by enhancing blood and lymphatic circulation and red blood cell production.

Respiratory system Enhances immunity; wards off infections, fevers, colds, flu, coughs, bronchitis and chest infections. • Relaxes bronchi in asthma.

Musculoskeletal system Anti-inflammatory and depurative for arthritis, osteomyelitis, rheumatism, lupus and rheumatism.

Immune system Antibacterial, antifungal and antiviral; helpful in herpes, flu and colds. • Lapachol has antioxidant, anticoagulant, antiviral, anti-inflammatory, antibacterial, antimalarial and anticancer properties. • May inhibit the growth of tumours by preventing cancer cells from using oxygen. • Useful for allergies and chronic fatigue.

Skin Helpful in skin disease, including eczema, psoriasis, ulcers, infections, candida, athlete's foot, herpes, impetigo, boils and acne.

Externally Applied to skin infections, eczema, psoriasis, cuts and sores and skin cancers.

CAUTION Avoid in pregnancy and blood-clotting disorders.

Drug interactions Avoid with anticoagulants.

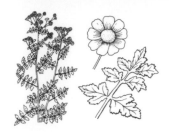
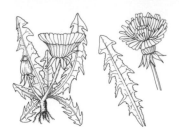

Tanacetum parthenium
Feverfew

An attractive perennial with aromatic leaves and daisy flowers that are loved by bees. So named because of its ability to bring down fevers. It is an excellent remedy for headaches and migraine. As prevention the leaves can be eaten daily in a sandwich or with other food.

Family Asteraceae

Parts used Aerial parts

Actions Diaphoretic, relaxant, uterine stimulant, anti-inflammatory, antihistamine, digestive bitter, nerve tonic, analgesic, depurative, decongestant, cholagogue.

Digestion Enhances appetite and digestion and allays nausea and vomiting. • Clears heat and toxins. • Bitter liver tonic. • Reduces symptoms associated with sluggish liver, such as lethargy, irritability, headaches and migraines.

Mental and emotional Nerve tonic; relaxes tension, lifts depression and promotes sleep. • Relieves nerve pain in shingles, trigeminal neuralgia and sciatica. • Used for oversensitivity to pain, irritability and anger. • Traditionally used for convulsions and fretful children.

Respiratory system Hot infusion increases perspiration and reduces fevers. It is decongestant and clears catarrh and sinusitis. • Used for asthma, migraine and other allergies such as hay fever due to its sesquiterpene lactones, which inhibit the release of prostaglandins and histamine. • Indicated in dizziness and tinnitus.

Musculoskeletal system Clears toxins and heat; useful anti-inflammatory for arthritis.

Externally The fresh plant is used on insect stings and bites to relieve pain and swelling. • Dilute tincture can be used as a lotion to repel insects and for spots and boils.

CAUTION Avoid during pregnancy. The fresh leaves may cause mouth ulcers.

Taraxacum officinale
Dandelion

Dandelion is a native of many Parts of Europe and Asia. The young leaves are traditionally eaten in the spring as a bitter detoxifying tonic to cleanse the body of wastes from the heavy, clogging food and more sedentary habits of winter.

Family Asteraceae

Parts used Leaf, root

Actions Digestive, bitter tonic, diuretic, mild laxative, cholagogue, depurative, anti-inflammatory.

Digestion Bitter digestive and liver tonic; enhances appetite and digestion, increases the flow of digestive juices and aids absorption. • Supports the liver as a major detoxifying organ; recommended in liver and gall bladder problems, hepatitis and problems associated with sluggish liver such as tiredness, irritability, headaches and skin problems. • The root is mildly laxative.

Immune system The root is anti-inflammatory; used for arthritis and rheumatism. • May increase insulin secretion from the pancreas; helpful in diabetes.

Urinary system The leaves are diuretic; useful in water retention, cellulite and urinary tract infections. Their high potassium content replaces that lost through increased urination. • Dissolve stones and gravel. • Improves the elimination of uric acid; useful remedy for gout.

Skin Detoxifying bitter tonic, increasing the elimination of toxins and wastes through the liver and kidneys, cleansing the blood and clearing the skin. For spots, acne, boils and abscesses.

Externally White juice from the stems can be applied to warts. • Infusion of the leaves and flowers is used for skin complaints.

CAUTION Avoid in obstruction of bile ducts and gall bladder. Milky latex in the leaves can cause dermatitis.

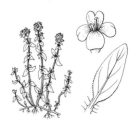
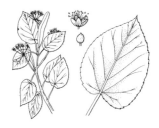

Thymus vulgaris
Thyme

An intensely aromatic small evergreen shrub native to the Mediterranean, found growing wild on warm, dry, rocky banks and heaths.

Family Lamiaceae

Parts used Flowering aerial parts

Actions Antispasmodic, astringent, digestive, antiseptic, antibacterial, decongestant, circulatory stimulan, relaxant, immunostimulant, antioxidant.

Digestion Enhances appetite and digestion and stimulates the liver. Used for indigestion, poor appetite, anaemia, liver and gall bladder complaints. • Flavonoids have relaxing effects and relieve wind, colic, IBS and spastic colon. • Astringent tannins protect the gut from irritation and reduce diarrhoea.

Circulation Warming stimulant; prevents chilblains and combats the effects of cold in winter.

Mental and emotional Strengthening tonic for physical and mental exhaustion. • Relieves tension, anxiety and depression.

Respiratory system For colds, sore throats, flu and chest infections. • Relieves asthma, whooping cough.

Immune system Volatile oils have powerful antibacterial and antifungal effects. They support the body's fight against infections, particularly in the respiratory, digestive and genitourinary systems. • Anti-inflammatory, possibly by inhibition of prostaglandin synthesis. • Antioxidant, protecting against degenerative problems. Increases longevity.

Urinary system Diuretic; relieves water retention.

Reproductive system Antispasmodic for dysmenorrhea. • Antimicrobial for infections such as candida and salpingitis.

Externally Used in liniments for aching joints, muscular pain and to disinfect cuts and wounds. • Gargle used for sore throats; and douche for vaginal infections.

CAUTION Avoid large amounts in pregnancy.

Tilia europaea
Lime flower

A deciduous tree native to Europe, western Asia and North America with a profusion of creamy flowers that make a delicious tea to reduce anxiety and fevers.

Family Tiliaceae

Parts used Flower

Actions Antispasmodic, thymoleptic, cholagogue, emollient, expectorant, hypotensive, sedative, stomachic, vasodilator, demulcent, diaphoretic, diuretic, ophthalmic, vermifuge (root).

Digestion Soothes and relaxes the gut; for digestive complaints associated with anxiety such as wind, colic, indigestion, diarrhoea, heartburn and acidity. • Roots act as a vermifuge for worms.

Circulation Antispasmodic; opens the arteries, reduces hypertension. • Protects blood vessel walls by reducing cholesterol build-up and hardening of the arteries. • Useful for migraine. • Diaphoretic; increases blood flow to the periphery. Reduces fevers. • A decoction of the roots and the bark has been used in the treatment of internal haemorrhaging.

Mental and emotional Antispasmodic and sedative; relieves tension, anxiety, insomnia, pain, nervous headaches, migraine, restlessness and agitation. Calms exam nerves.

Respiratory system Decongestant and soothing expectorant for feverish colds, flu, catarrh, irritating coughs, bronchitis and asthma.

Urinary system Soothing diuretic; clears toxins via the kidneys, relieves cystitis, urethritis and frequent urination due to nerves.

Externally Infusion of leaves used as an eyewash; poultice for burns and scalds. • Infusion of the flowers is applied to spots, acne, boils, burns and rashes to clear heat and irritation. • Gargle used for mouth ulcers. • Added to baths to calm restless children.

CAUTION Large doses may cause nausea. Excess use may damage the heart.

Tinospora cordifolia
Guduchi

A vigorous creeper that grows in the forests of India and is a renowned rejuvenative in Ayurvedic medicine.

Family Menispermaceae

Parts used Stem, leaf

Actions Adaptogen, digestive, astringent, anti-fungal, rejuvenative, alterative, diuretic, cholagogue, anti-inflammatory, antioxidant, probiotic, vermifuge.

Digestion Enhances energy by improving appetite, digestion and absorption. • Reduces inflammation in acidity, gastritis, peptic ulcers, nausea and vomiting. • Re-establishes gut flora. Dispels worms. Antifungal; helpful in candida. • Relieves constipation and clears toxins. • Used for chronic hepatitis and toxic damage. Aids liver tissue regeneration. • Stabilizes blood sugar.

Circulation Reduces bleeding tendency such as in bleeding gums and haemorrhoids. Useful in anaemia. • Lowers harmful cholesterol.

Mental and emotional Adaptogenic; increases resistance to emotional and physical stress. • Increases energy yet relaxes tension.

Respiratory system Helps resolve infections and catarrhal congestion. Indicated in coughs, colds, flu, sinusitis and allergies such as hay fever and asthma.

Musculoskeletal system Anti-inflammatory for joint problems; used for gout and with Ginger for arthritis.

Immune system Antioxidant and antitumour activity; reduces side effects of radiotherapy and chemotherapy. • Stimulates antibody production and macrophage function. Improves resistance to infection. • Lowers fevers.

Urinary system Aids elimination of uric acid; helpful for arthritis and gout.

Skin Clears skin problems such as eczema and psoriasis.

CAUTION Excessive doses can inhibit B vitamin assimilation and can cause nausea.

Trifolium pratense
Red clover

A perennial native herb to Europe, North America and western Asia, found growing wild in meadows.

Family Fabaceae

Parts used Flowering top

Actions Alterative, antioxidant, antispasmodic, antitumour, diuretic, expectorant, sedative.

Circulation Helps prevent hypertension. Coumarins may affect platelet activity and reduce lipids.

Respiratory system Antispasmodic and expectorant for catarrh, whooping cough, dry coughs, bronchitis and asthma.

Immune system Traditionally used as a detoxifying herb for cancer of the breast, lung and lymphatic system. Flavone glycosides have been shown to inhibit cancer by inhibiting angiogenesis and cancer cell adhesion. • Indicated in chronic degenerative diseases and lymphatic congestion.

Musculoskeletal system Beneficial to post-menopausal women. • Used for arthritis and gout.

Reproductive system Flavone glycosides increase follicle-stimulating hormones and are oestrogenic; useful for menopausal complaints such as hot flushes, night sweats and insomnia. • Benefits lymphatic system; helpful in mastitis. • Helps prevent prostate problems. • Traditionally used for breast and ovarian cancer.

Skin Clears toxins; helps resolve skin complaints, especially eczema and psoriasis.

Externally Poultices are applied to skin problems and cancerous growths.

CAUTION Avoid in bleeding disorders, pregnancy and breast-feeding. Diseased clover, even if no symptoms of disease are visible, can contain toxic alkaloids.

Drug interactions Use with caution with anticoagulants and contraceptives.

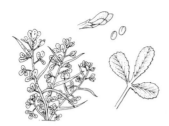
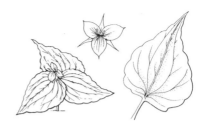

Trigonella foenum-graecum
Fenugreek

Fenugreek is a member of the pea family and native to the Mediterranean, Ukraine and India. Highly nutritious, the seeds are well known as a cooking spice and are used in Africa as a coffee substitute.

Family Fabaceae

Parts used Seed

Actions Digestive, laxative, demulcent, emollient, expectorant, diuretic, antiviral, antihypertensive, hypoglycaemic, hypocholesterolaemic, oestrogenic.

Digestion Enhances appetite, digestion and absorption. • Mucilagin coats the gut lining, protecting it from irritation and inflammation in gastritis, acid indigestion and peptic ulcers. • Not absorbed, so adds fibre and acts as a bulk laxative in constipation. • Possesses hypoglycaemic activity by delaying gastric emptying, slowing carbohydrate absorption and inhibiting glucose transport. It may also increase insulin receptors in red blood cells and improve glucose utilization in peripheral tissues.

Circulation Lowers harmful cholesterol and triglycerides. • Reduces blood pressure and inhibits clotting; helps to prevent heart and arterial disease.

Respiratory system Expectorant and immune-enhancing for chronic coughs and bronchitis. • Antiviral.

Urinary system Diuretic; aids elimination of toxins via the kidneys.

Reproductive system Diosgenin is used to create semisynthetic forms of oestrogen. Can enlarge breast size. • Reduces menopausal symptoms such as hot flushes, night sweats, vaginal dryness and insomnia. • Stimulates milk flow in nursing mothers. Externally Decoction used as a lotion for boils, ulcers and eczema.

CAUTION Avoid in pregnancy.

Drug interactions Use with caution with antidiabetic and anticoagulant drugs.

Trillium erectum
Beth root

A beautiful woodland plant native to North America, renowned among Native American tribes for lessening pain during childbirth and preventing post-partum bleeding.

Family Trilliaceae

Parts used Rhizome, root

Actions Astringent, partus praeparator, antiseptic, antifungal, uterine tonic, hormone regulator, antihaemorrhagic, alterative, expectorant.

Digestion Astringent; tones and protects the gut lining, reducing inflammation and bleeding. Recommended in inflammatory bowel problems, diarrhoea, dysentery and bleeding.

Respiratory system Astringent and expectorant; dries up excess secretions and reduces catarrh. Helpful in catarrhal coughs, asthma, chronic lung problems and haemoptysis.

Urinary system Used for haematuria.

Reproductive system Traditionally used to induce childbirth, stimulate contractions and reduce pain. • Regulates hormones and relieves menstrual problems. • Astringent; constricts blood vessels. Used for fibroids, heavy bleeding, dysfunctional uterine bleeding and post-partum haemorrhage. • Reduces perimenopausal flooding and menopausal symptoms. • Relieves sore nipples. • Aphrodisiac.

Externally Lotion used to reduce bleeding speed, healing of ulcers, for inflammatory skin problems, haemorrhoids and varicose veins, tumours, insect bites and stings. • Antiseptic/antifungal douche used for vaginal infections such as candida and trichomonas; reduces discharges.

CAUTION Avoid during pregnancy and gastric reflux.

Drug interactions May decrease the effects of cardiac glycosides.

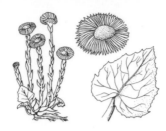
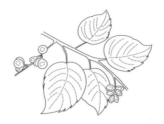

Tussilago farfara
Coltsfoot

A perennial herb that grows throughout Europe, in North Africa and western and northern Asia in hedgerows, woodland and meadows. Its bright yellow flowers resembling dandelions appear before the leaves. It is famous as a remedy for respiratory problems, traditionally used in cough syrups or candied and sucked as a sweet.

Family Asteraceae

Parts used Leaf, flower

Actions Antispasmodic, anti-inflammatory, emollient, bronchodilator, demulcent, antitussive, diuretic, astringent, diaphoretic, expectorant, digestive.

Digestion Improves digestion and appetite. Soothes irritation of the gut lining.

Respiratory system Soothing, anti-inflammatory and expectorant for colds, catarrh, sore throats, tonsillitis, dry, persistent coughs, bronchitis and asthma. Particularly useful for relieving coughing in chronic emphysema and silicosis. • Rich in zinc it promotes tissue repair; indicated for susceptibility to coughs and chest infections due to damage to respiratory system following infection or from smoking. • Antispasmodic effects are helpful for relieving bronchospasm in asthma.

Immune system Enhances immunity; helps resolve infection and prevents platelet aggregation.

Urinary system Soothes irritation and inflammation; used for cystitis and urethritis.

Externally Poultice of flowers soothes and promotes healing of skin disorders such as eczema, ulcers, sores, bites and other inflammation.

CAUTION Contains traces of liver-affecting pyrrolizidine alkaloids (largely destroyed when the plant is boiled to make a decoction). Potentially toxic in large doses. Take for a maximum of 28 days at a time. Avoid in liver disease, pregnancy and breast-feeding, and in children under 6.

Ulmus fulva
Slippery elm

A deciduous tree growing in Canada and the USA. The inner bark from trees that are at least ten years old was used by Native Americans to soothe an irritated digestive system and as a poultice for wounds and ulcers.

Family Ulmaceae

Parts used Inner bark, generally as powder

Actions Demulcent, emollient, nutritive, antitussive, antioxidant, anti-inflammatory, diuretic, expectorant, laxative, rejuvenative, probiotic.

Digestion Polysaccharide molecules expand in water and create a gruel that coats the gut lining and soothes pain in inflammatory conditions, acid reflux, heartburn, nausea, gastritis, colitis, peptic ulcers, IBS, diverticulitis and leaky gut syndrome. • Good bulk laxative for constipation. • Enhances growth of normal gut flora. • Nourishing food when weak, particularly good for infants and elderly, as it is easy to digest.

Respiratory system Moistens and reduces heat irritation and inflammation in the throat and chest, relieves catarrh and dry coughs. • Traditionally used for bronchitis, pneumonia and pleurisy. • Relaxes throat and bronchi; used for sore throats, hoarseness, laryngitis, pharyngitis, asthma and whooping cough.

Musculoskeletal system Rich in calcium for strengthening bones and promoting healing.

Immune system Anti-inflammatory, enhances immunity. • Soothing and strengthening when recovering from illness or undergoing chemotherapy. Ingredient of the renowned anticancer formula Essiac.

Urinary system Soothes the lining of the urinary tract; reduces pain and inflammation in cystitis.

Externally Used as a poultice for drawing out toxins in boils, abscesses and varicose ulcers. • Applied to wounds, burns and inflammation to reduce swelling and pain.

Drug interactions Separate from medicines taken by 2 hours; may inhibit absorption.

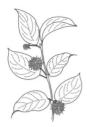
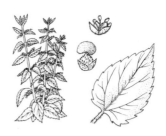

Uncaria tomentosa
Cat's claw

A climbing vine native to the Amazonian jungle, where it has been famous as a remedy for infections and inflammatory conditions.

Family Rubiaceae

Parts used Bark, root, leaf

Actions Immune enhancing, anti-inflammatory, antioxidant, antitumour, antimicrobial, diuretic.

Digestion Strengthens the gut in Crohn's disease, inflammatory bowel disorders, diverticulitis and leaky gut syndrome. • Used in gastritis, ulcers, diarrhoea, dysentery and candidiasis. • Enhances liver function.

Circulation Inhibits blood platelet aggregation, strengthens blood vessels and helps prevent strokes.

Respiratory system Gives immune support in asthma, bronchitis and hay fever.

Musculoskeletal system Anti-inflammatory for osteo- and rheumatoid arthritis, lupus, bursitis and gout.

Immune system Oxidole alkaloids stimulate immunity by enhancing the activity of phagocytes, macrophages, lymphocytes and leucocytes. Used for chronic immune deficiency and HIV, chronic fatigue, allergies and tendency to infections. • Slows growth of leukaemia cells. Used as a complement to cancer treatments; protects against effects of chemotherapy.

Urinary system Used for urinary tract infections.

Reproductive system Regulates the menstrual cycle; relieves PMS. • Helpful in prostatitis.

Eyes Reduces inflammatory problems such as conjunctivitis and iritis.

Externally Lotions/creams used for acne, herpes, shingles, athlete's foot, haemorrhoids and cuts. • Eye lotion used for conjunctivitis.

CAUTION Avoid in pregnancy.

Drug interactions Use cautiously with immunosuppressive drugs.

Urtica dioica
Nettle

This perennial grows throughout Europe, Asia, North Africa and North America. It is nutritious, rich in vitamins A and C, and minerals.

Family Urticaceae

Parts used Aerial parts of young plants, root, seed

Actions Alterative, astringent, haemostatic, diuretic, blood building, antihistamine.

Digestion Astringent tannins protect the gut lining from irritation and infection. • Relieves diarrhoea and flatulence. • Stimulates liver and kidney function and clears toxins. • Reduces blood sugar. • Seeds improve thyroid function and reduce goitre.

Respiratory system Clears catarrh in coughs, bronchitis, hay fever and asthma. • Seeds/fresh juice used for fevers and lung disorders.

Immune system Detoxifying. • Antihistamine for allergies such as asthma and hay fever. • Flavonoids have immunostimulatory effects. • Antibacterial activity against Staphylococcus aureus and S. albus.

Reproductive system Stimulates milk production in nursing mothers. • Regulates periods and reduces heavy bleeding. • Rich in iron.

Urinary system Diuretic; relieves fluid retention, cystitis and urethritis. • Softens stones and gravel. • Helps prevent bed-wetting and incontinence. • Enhances excretion of uric acid; good for gout and arthritis. • Root used for benign prostatic hypertrophy.

Skin Depurative and anti-inflammatory; clears skin in eczema, urticaria and other chronic skin problems.

Externally Fresh juice/tea used for cuts, wounds, haemorrhoids, burns and scalds, bites/stings, including nettle sting.

CAUTION Avoid in oedema from impaired cardiac or renal function.

Drug interactions Avoid with diuretics and antihypertensives.

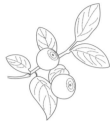

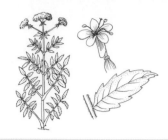

Vaccinium myrtillus
Blueberry/Bilberry

A perennial shrub, native to Europe, bearing black shiny berries, which are a potent source of antioxidants.

Family Ericaceae

Parts used Fruit, leaf

Actions Antioxidant, anti-inflammatory, astringent, vasoprotective, antispasmodic, diuretic, rejuvenative.

Digestion Increases gastric mucous. Reduces inflammation of the stomach and intestinal lining, and protects the gut lining against excess acid. • Leaves are a traditional remedy for diabetes, diarrhoea, vomiting, typhoid and stomach cramps. • Berries reduce blood sugar and are mildly laxative and astringent; relieve constipation and diarrhoea.

Circulation Antioxidant; enhances circulation and protects arteries from free radical damage. Useful in Raynaud's disease, capillary fragility, bleeding gums, spider veins, haemorrhoids, varicose veins and venous insufficiency. • Anthocyanosides stabilize collagen and help rebuild capillaries. • Reduces platelet aggregation, prevents clots and protects against heart attacks and strokes without the risk of increased bleeding.

Musculoskeletal system Antioxidant and anti-inflammatory, stabilizes collagen; helpful in arthritis.

Urinary system Anti-inflammatory; and diuretic used for bladder infections and stones.

Reproductive system Antispasmodic; relieves dysmenorrhoea.

Eyes Antioxidant action prevents free radical damage that can cause cataracts and macular degeneration. • Used for diabetic or hypertensive retinopathy; strengthens collagen and protects eye tissue against glaucoma and eyestrain. • Regenerates rhodopsin, a pigment found in the retina that is vital to good night vision.

Externally Promotes healing; useful after surgery. • Mouthwash used for inflammation of the mouth and gums; gargle for sore throats.

Valeriana officinalis
Valerian

A perennial wild plant with pretty pink flowers native to Europe, Asia and North America. The root is highly pungent with a smell that is disliked by many but loved by cats.

Family Valerianaceae

Parts used Root, rhizome

Actions Anxiolytic, sedative, hypnotic, anodyne, anthelmintic, antibacterial, antispasmodic, astringent, bitter, carminative, diaphoretic, diuretic, hypotensive, restorative, stomachic, tonic.

Digestion Antispasmodic and sedative. Relaxes tension and spasm in stress-related problems such as dyspepsia, intestinal colic and IBS.

Circulation Lowers blood pressure. • Increases blood flow to the heart. • Calms nervous palpitations.

Mental and emotional Well-known sedative and nerve tonic; valepotriates are mainly responsible for its calming effects. Excellent for anxiety, nervous tension, agitation, panic attacks, irritability, insomnia, nervous headaches and exhaustion. • Strengthens and calms the heart. Relieves nervous palpitations. • Relaxing to smooth muscle; useful for stress-related disorders such as muscle tension, colic, IBS, period pain and headaches. • Useful in treatment of addiction (tobacco or tranquillizer), chronic aggression and ADD. • Historically an esteemed remedy for epilepsy, hysteria, convulsions, migraine, headaches and most nerve problems; used in World War I for shell shock and nerve strain caused by air raids.

Respiratory system Antispasmodic for paroxysmal coughs and croup.

Reproductive system Antispasmodic for period pain.

CAUTION Avoid prolonged use. Excessive doses may cause headaches, muscle spasm, insomnia or palpitations.

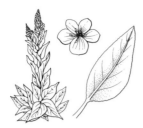

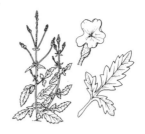

Verbascum thapsus
Mullein

This impressive biennial, with tall spikes of yellow flowers is native to Europe, Asia and North Africa.

Family Scrophulariaceae

Parts used Leaf, flower, root

Actions Expectorant, astringent, sedative, demulcent, decongestant, anodyne, antispasmodic.

Digestion Soothes the gut, eases peptic ulcers and curbs diarrhoea.

Mental and emotional Painkiller for headaches, neuralgia, arthritis and rheumatism; encourages sleep. • Specifically for earache; applied locally and taken internally for catarrhal deafness, tinnitus, ear infections, wax accumulation and head pain caused by ear congestion. • Relieves anxiety, nervous palpitations, heart irregularities, cramps and nervous colic. • Astringent properties curb nervous diarrhoea. • Root decoction was a traditional remedy for toothache and convulsions.

Respiratory system Soothing expectorant for harsh, dry coughs, sore throats and inflammatory conditions such as pharyngitis, tracheitis, bronchitis and bronchiectasis. Traditional remedy for TB, whooping cough and pleurisy. • Relaxing and antiseptic; relieves colds, flu, asthma, croup and chest infections. • Decongestant; clears phlegm, sinusitis and hay fever.

Immune system Enhances immunity. • Anti-inflammatory; relieves the pain of swollen glands and mumps. • Antibacterial and antiviral activity against influenza strains and herpes simplex.

Urinary system Soothing diuretic for burning and frequency of cystitis, and fluid retention. • Increases the elimination of toxins; useful for arthritis, rheumatism and gout.

Externally Compress of leaves used for painful joints and muscles, asthma, headaches, swollen glands and mumps. • Speeds healing of wounds, burns, sores, ulcers and piles. • Mullein oil from the flowers used as eardrops for earache and eczema of the outer ear.

Verbena officinalis
Vervain

Native to Europe, this perennial has attractive spikes of mauve flowers in summer and is found growing wild from Denmark to North Africa and western Asia to the Himalayas.

Family Verbenaceae

Parts used Aerial parts

Actions Thymoleptic, nerve tonic, antioxidant, analgesic, antibacterial, anticoagulant, antispasmodic, antitumor, astringent, birthing aid, depurative, diaphoretic, tonic, hepatic, sedative.

Digestion Enhances appetite and improves absorption. May be useful in anorexia, hypochloridia and indigestion. • Bitters stimulate the liver and relieve headaches, lethargy, irritability and constipation. Used for liver disorders and gallstones. • Root is astringent; used for diarrhoea and dysentery.

Mental and emotional Excellent tonic; calms irritability and anxiety, lifts depression and supports the body during stress. For stress-related symptoms such as headaches, indigestion, insomnia, high blood pressure, muscle pain and nervous exhaustion. • Helpful for convalescence after stress or illness and in chronic fatigue syndrome. • Verbenin is thought to block sympathetic innervation of the heart, blood vessels and intestines.

Immune system Taken hot it reduces fevers.

Urinary system Taken cool it has a diuretic and detoxifying action; useful for fluid retention and gout.

Reproductive system Regulates periods and relieves PMS. • Enhances contractions during childbirth. • Enhances milk supply in nursing mothers; for insufficient lactation associated with stress.

Externally Astringent mouthwash used for bleeding gums and mouth ulcers. • Lotions used for cuts, insect bites, eczema, sores and neuralgia.

CAUTION Do not take simultaneously with mineral supplements. Avoid during pregnancy.

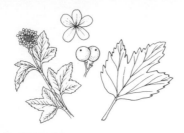

Viburnum opulus

Cramp bark

Native to Europe, North America and northern Asia, this striking tree, with its bright red berries, was prized among Native American and pioneer women to prevent miscarriage and relieve period pains.

Family Caprifoliaceae

Parts used Bark, stem bark

Actions Antispasmodic, hypotensive, peripheral vasodilator, sedative, carminative, astringent, partus praeparator, anodyne.

Digestion Relaxes tension and spasm. Relieves stress-related disorders such as colic, nausea, wind, abdominal cramps and IBS.

Circulation Dilates the arteries, reduces blood pressure. • Used for palpitations and angina. • Releases tension in arteries, relieves leg cramps, helpful in Raynaud's syndrome.

Musculoskeletal system Used as a general muscle relaxant for voluntary and involuntary muscular cramp and tension. Famous as a remedy for leg cramps. • Used for tension headaches.productive system • Uterine sedative and tonic. Aesculetin and scopoletin have a powerful antispasmodic action, relieving cramps. Salicin is a good pain reliever. Used in spasmodic dysmenorrhoea for bearing-down pain, back and thigh pain, heavy bleeding, endometriosis, threatened/repeated miscarriage and to prepare for labour. • Helps prevent uterine irritability, over-strong contractions, false labour pains and afterpains. • Prevents excessive menstrual flow during the menopause. • Used as an antispasmodic for benign prostatic hypertrophy. Astringent action is helpful in prolapse.

Respiratory system Relaxes spasm in bronchi; useful for harsh irritating coughs and asthma as an adjuvant.

CAUTION The fresh berries are poisonous. Avoid with anticoagulant drugs.

Viburnum prunifolium

Black haw

A small deciduous tree native to North America, where its medicinal benefits were taught by the Native American to the settlers. It was primarily used as a remedy for women, for preparing the uterus for childbirth, to relieve pain and reduce bleeding.

Family Caprifoliaceae

Parts used Bark, root

Actions Uterine antispasmodic, astringent, bronchodilator, hypotensive, diuretic, sedative, partus praeparator.

Digestion Relieves the nausea of pregnancy. • Used for abdominal spasms, especially chronic hiccups, hiatus hernia and gastric or intestinal cramps and diarrhoea.

Circulation Lowers arterial blood pressure. • Useful for venospasm and as an adjunctive treatment for mild to moderate hypertension. • Used for asthma.

Mental and emotional Helps calm anxiety, particularly when related to miscarriage.

Reproductive system Amphoteric effect on uterine muscles, toning over-relaxed muscles while relaxing tension in muscles causing spasm and pain. • Scopoletin and aesculetin have both been shown to have a sedative effect on the uterus. Prepares the uterus for childbirth. • Improves circulation to the uterus and ovaries and promotes nutrition to the pelvic area. • Relieves dysmenorrhoea with scanty flow. • It can be used for threatened/repeated miscarriage and nocturnal leg cramps during pregnancy. • Eases childbirth, relieves false pains and labour pains and prevents post-partum haemorrhage. • Helps normal involution of the womb after childbirth. • Strengthening tonic after miscarriage.

CAUTION Use cautiously in cases of kidney stones.

Drug interactions Avoid with anticoagulants such as heparin and warfarin.

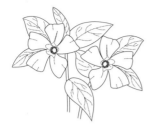

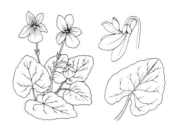

Vinca major and V. minor
Greater and Lesser periwinkle

Evergreen perennials with blue windmill-shaped flowers that grow wild throughout Europe. The flowers and leaves were traditionally chewed to relieve toothache.

Family Apocynaceae

Parts used Flower, leaf

Actions Astringent, sedative, hypotensive, hypoglycaemic, thymoleptic.

Digestion Astringent tannins curb diarrhoea and dysentery, protect the gut wall from irritation and infection and stop bleeding. • Healing remedy for heartburn, gastritis, peptic ulcers and flatulence. • May help regulate blood sugar and prevent diabetes.

Circulation Improves blood flow to the brain; recommended in cerebral arteriosclerosis and after stroke. • Reduces high blood pressure and helps prevent atherosclerosis.

Mental and emotional Reduces tension, relieves anxiety, lifts depression and SAD, clears the mind and boosts energy levels.

Respiratory system Astringent; clears chronic catarrh and phlegm.

Immune system Vinca rosea (now Catharanthus roseus)/Madagascan periwinkle was discovered in the 1920s to reduce blood sugar in diabetics, and hailed as a possible substitute for insulin. Lesser and Greater periwinkles have also been used for diabetes. • Alkaloids vinblastine and vincristine in Vinca rosea have been extensively used to treat malignant tumours, leukaemia and Hodgkin's disease.

Reproductive system Reduces excessive menstrual bleeding and vaginal discharge.

Externally Used to make vaginal douches for discharges; lotions for haemorrhoids, varicose veins and skin problems such as acne and cradle cap; mouthwashes and gargles for mouth ulcers, tonsillitis and sore throats. • Chewed to relieve toothache and combat bleeding gums.

Viola odorata
Sweet violet

Native to Asia and Europe, the sweet violet was traditionally woven into garlands to cool anger, cure headaches and hangovers and induce sleep. Hippocrates recommended it for melancholia, bad eyesight and inflammation of the chest.

Family Violaceae

Parts used Flower, leaf

Actions Expectorant, antitumour, demulcent, diaphoretic, alterative, antifungal, anti-inflammatory, antiseptic, antiscorbutic, astringent, emollient, febrifuge, laxative, nutritive, restorative.

Digestion Soothes irritation and inflamation in the gut. • Gentle laxative.

Mental and emotional Recommended for grief and heartbreak and to improve memory. • Eases headache from lack of sleep and helps moderate anger.

Respiratory system Soothing expectorant for harsh, irritating coughs and chest infections, pleurisy, chronic bronchitis, tonsillitis, asthma and chronic catarrh; popular in children's cough syrup. • Hot tea brings down fevers and clears colds and congestion.

Musculoskeletal system Cools heat and inflammation; salicylates useful for arthritis.

Immune system In Traditional Chinese Medicine used for hot swellings, cysts and tumours. • Used in the treatment of cancer (breast, lung, digestive tract, skin, throat and tongue). • Deters infection.

Urinary system Soothes inflamed and painful conditions such as cystitis, trichomonas, urethritis and urinary tract infections.

Externally Compress or poultice used to treat boils, conjunctivitis, breast cysts, cancers and haemorrhoids. • A cloth soaked in violet tea can be applied to the back of the neck to treat headaches.

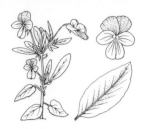

Viola tricolor
Wild pansy

Native to temperate parts of Europe, this charming plant was historically renowned for its ability to clear stubborn skin problems. It is often called heartsease because of its ancient reputation for curing affairs of the heart. Hippocrates used it as a cordial to lift the spirits and treat heart conditions.

Family Violaceae

Parts used Leaf, flower

Actions Anti-inflammatory, antirheumatic, expectorant, diuretic, alterative, laxative, antiallergenic, hypotensive, demulcent, decongestant.

Circulation Enhances circulation, reduces blood pressure, strengthens blood vessels and helps prevent arteriosclerosis.

Respiratory system Soothing and expectorant properties useful for inflammatory chest problems, bronchitis, harsh, irritating coughs, whooping cough, asthma and croup. • The saponins account for its expectorant action, while its mucilage content soothes the chest. • Taken hot it relieves catarrhal congestion and brings down fevers.

Immune system Used to reduce heat and inflammation and clear skin conditions. Helps clear chronic skin disorders with purulent sticky discharge, moist eczema, milk crust and ringworm. • Traditionally used for skin cancer, seborrheic skin disease, acne, impetigo, pruritus vulvae and cradle cap. • Salicylates are helpful for treating arthritis and gout.

Urinary system Soothing diuretic; relieves cystitis and fluid retention, and clears toxins. • Relieves painful and frequent urination.

Externally Lotion used for seborrheic skin disease, acne, impetigo, pruritus vulvae and cradle cap.

CAUTION Avoid if allergic to salicylates.

Drug interactions May increase actions of salicylates (aspirin).

Viscum album
Mistletoe

An evergreen partial parasite native to Europe, North Africa and Asia, which draws nourishment and medicinal constituents from the host deciduous tree. When used medicinally, it is usually taken from apple trees.

Family Loranthaceae

Parts used Leaf, young twig

Actions Vasodilator, hypotensive, diuretic, antispasmodic, immunostimulant, antitumour, narcotic, sedative.

Circulation Regulates heart and blood pressure, normalizes pulse and calms rapid heart and nervous palpitations. • Dilates arteries. • Useful for angina and helpful for arteriosclerotic narrowing of the arteries. • Strengthens capillary walls, improves circulation and relaxes muscles. • Relieves headaches due to high blood pressure. • Useful for varicose veins.

Mental and emotional Sedative, muscle relaxant and nerve tonic; used for epilepsy, convulsions, panic attacks, nervous debility, tense, aching muscles, anxiety, insomnia, cramps, nervous headaches, migraines and vertigo. • Increases resilience to stress.

Immune system Enhances immunity, specifically the function of the thymus gland and spleen, accelerating antibody production; used for lowered immunity, chronic candida, ME and HIV. • Cytotoxic alkaloids and lectins may have antitumour effects; the 'viscum therapy' of injecting fresh mistletoe extracts in cancer originated in Switzerland based on the findings of Rudolf Steiner. • Aids recovery of energy, health and appetite after orthodox cancer treatment. • May have anti-inflammatory effect in gout. • An injectable form of mistletoe lectins has been used to reduce the signs and symptoms of hepatitis.

CAUTION Raw mistletoe is toxic, as are the berries. Only use under professional guidance and in small doses. May cause temporary numbness, vomiting and reduced heart rate. Avoid during pregnancy.

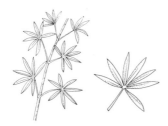

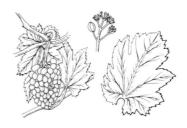

Vitex agnus castus
Chaste tree

An attractive shrub, native to seashores of Europe, North Africa and Asia, with long spikes of mauve flowers and highly aromatic seeds. Its name derives from its reputation for calming sexual desires, particularly in men.

Family Verbenaceae

Parts used Berry

Actions Carminative, diaphoretic, anaphrodisiac, antiandrogenic, aromatic, diuretic, emmenagogue, febrifuge, ophthalmic, phytoprogesteronic, sedative, stomachic.

Urinary system Diuretic; relieves fluid retention, particularly accompanying PMS.

Reproductive system Acts on the pituitary gland to regulate the production of follicle-stimulating hormone, luteinizing hormone and prolactin. This leads to an increase in progesterone production during the second half of the cycle, balancing hormones that regulate menstruation and fertility. • Relieves symptoms associated with high oestrogen and low progesterone, such as migraines, breast tenderness, bloating, mood swings, cramps, fluid retention, constipation, herpes (related to menses), premenstrual acne, PMS and threatened miscarriage. • Taken over 3–6 months it regulates menstrual cycle and relieves painful periods, fibrocystic breast disease, PMS, acne and endometriosis. • Reduces prolactin secretion; useful for benign breast problems, fibroids, and prostatic hypertrophy. • Enhances fertility and remedies amenorrhoea and menorrhagia caused by corpus luteum insufficiency. • Useful in polycystic ovary syndrome, endometriosis, cysts (in breasts, ovaries and uterus) and threatened miscarriage. • Stimulates milk flow in nursing mothers. • Used for menopausal symptoms such as hot flushes, vaginal dryness and depression. • Regulates menstrual cycle in women coming off birth control pills. • Beneficial after hysterectomy and childbirth.

Drug interactions Avoid with HRT or the contraceptive pill.

Vitis vinifera
Red grape

The common grape vine is native to the Mediterranean, central Europe and southwestern Asia.

Family Vitaceae

Parts used Seed and skin of fruit

Actions Antioxidant, astringent, collagen stabilizer, circulatory tonic, anti-inflammatory, probiotic.

Digestion Astringent tannins protect the gastrointestinal tract from irritation and inflammation. • Used in gastritis, ulcers and pancreatitis. • Essential fatty acids and tocopherols protect the liver and prevent the oxidation of vitamin E. • Helps regulate gut flora in dysbiosis.

Circulation Improves circulation and venous return; useful for peripheral vascular disease such as Raynaud's disease, venous insufficiency, varicose veins and haemorrhoids. • Strengthens blood vessel walls. Used for capillary fragility and diabetic and hypertensive retinopathy. • Protects collagen from degradation and reduces harmful cholesterol and blood pressure. • Inhibits platelet activity without prolonging bleeding. • Antioxidant; helps prevent cardiovascular disease.

Musculoskeletal system Reduces pain and inflammation in joints and protects synovial fluid and collagen.

Immune system Re-establishes normal bacterial population of the gut. • Antioxidants may protect against tumour formation especially in the breast, stomach, colon, prostate and lung. • Good after radiation therapy for cancer. • May help protect liver damage from toxins and chemotherapy.

Reproductive system Used for chloasma and congestive dysmenorrhoea.

Eyes Inhibits macular degeneration and diabetic retinopathy; improves nearsightedness.

Externally Strengthens connective tissue and promotes healing.

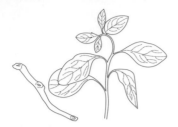
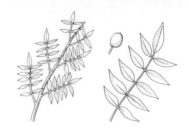

Withania somniferum
Ashwagandha/Winter cherry

Native to India, and one of the most important herbs in Ayurvedic medicine. As a restorative and rejuvenative it is esteemed as highly as Ginseng in Traditional Chinese Medicine.

Family Solanaceae

Parts used Root

Actions Sedative, antispasmodic, anticonvulsant, nerve tonic, diuretic, astringent, nutritive, rejuvenative, anti-inflammatory, anticancer, cardioprotective, hypotensive, adaptogen, antioxidant, aphrodisiac, immunomodulatory, thyroid balancing.

Mental and emotional Adaptogen; modifies the harmful effects of stress on mind and body. Engenders clarity of mind. Excellent for stress, anxiety, depression, overwork, panic attacks, nervous exhaustion and insomnia. • Used for behavioural problems, poor memory and concentration, ADHD and problems associated with drug abuse/addiction. • Used for problems associated with old age such as loss of energy and muscular strength, arthritis and insomnia.

Respiratory system Immune enhancing and antimicrobial; increases resistance to infections.

Immune system Anti-inflammatory for joint problems. • Decreases free radical damage and slows the ageing process. • Enhances immunity; used for chronic immune deficiency, fibromyalgia, HIV, autoimmune problems such as MS, ankylosing spondylitis, lupus and rheumatoid arthritis. • May inhibit the growth of cancers. • Supports the system during chemotherapy and radiation therapy.

GenitoUrinary system Used for urinary problems, dysmenorrhea, irregular and scanty periods and endometriosis. • Famous for infertility and as a male reproductive tonic.

Externally Oil used for arthritic joints, frozen shoulder and nerve pain such as sciatica, muscle spasm and back pain. • Used for wounds, sores and dry, itchy skin conditios.

CAUTION Avoid over 3 g daily in pregnancy.

Zanthoxylum americanum
Prickly ash

A tall shrub native to North America. It has warming and stimulating effects.

Family Rutaceae

Parts used Bark

Actions Circulatory stimulant, diaphoretic, alterative, analgesic, anthelmintic, antibacterial, anti-inflammatory, antispasmodic, astringent, emmenagogue, immunostimulant, digestive.

Digestion Improves digestion and absorption, and increases pancreas and liver function. • Used for constipation due to deficient secretions, colic, bloating and wind.

Circulation Increases blood flow to the periphery; used for chilblains, intermittent claudication, Raynaud's disease, Buerger's disease, cerebrovascular disease, varicose veins, haemorrhoids and leg cramps. • Prevents blood platelet aggregation and regulates blood pressure. • Stimulates lymphatic circulation. • Increases kidney output and cardiac function.

Mental and emotional Strengthening stimulant; used for debility and nervous exhaustion. • Helpful in neuralgia and restless leg syndrome.

Respiratory system Useful in chronic pharyngitis and post-nasal catarrh. • Diaphoretic when taken hot; helps resolve chills, colds, coughs, flu, fevers, sore throats.

Musculoskeletal system Alterative properties are helpful for osteoarthritis, rheumatism, gout and lumbago.

Immune system Enhances fight against infection and cancer. • Used as a capillary stimulant for resolving eruptive diseases such as measles and chickenpox.

Reproductive system Stimulates blood flow to the uterus; relieves uterine cramps and dysmenorrhoea.

CAUTION Avoid in pregnancy and with gastrointestinal inflammation.

Drug interactions Avoid with anticoagulants and antihypertensives.

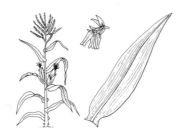 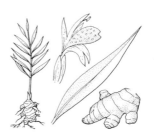

Zea mays
Corn silk

Corn silk is the yellow strands inside the husks of corn, harvested before pollination. Native to Central and South America, it is rich in nutrients and contains silicon, B vitamins, para-amino benzoic acid and small amounts of iron, zinc, potassium, vitamin K, calcium, magnesium and phosphorus. For best results use fresh.

Family Poaceae

Parts used Style, stigma

Actions Urinary demulcent, diuretic, liver tonic, hypoglycaemic, hypotensive, alterative, anti-inflammatory, antiseptic, tonic.

Digestion Stimulates bile flow from the liver and aids the liver's detoxifying work. • Helps regulate blood sugar.

Circulation Dilates arteries and reduces blood pressure and blood clotting time. • Good source of vitamin K; helps control bleeding, for example during childbirth.

Urinary system Demulcent diuretic for cystitis, dysuria, urethritis and bed-wetting. • Anti-inflammatory effects are useful in the treatment of acute and chronic prostatitis and inflammatory conditions of the bladder and kidneys. • Excellent for symptoms associated with benign enlargement of the prostate. • Reduces fluid retention and aids elimination of toxins and excess uric acid via the kidneys; helpful in gout and arthritis and chronic skin problems such as boils. • Helps to dissolve stones and gravel. • Useful in fluid retention associated with PMS.

Other Anti-inflammatory for arthritis, skin problems and for carpal tunnel syndrome.

Externally Applied powdered to soothe and speed healing of the skin.

CAUTION Avoid in corn allergies.

Zingiber officinale
Ginger

A wonderfully pungent spice native to South Asia. Its warming and energizing properties were mentioned in the writings of Confucius as early as 500 BCE.

Family Zingiberaceae

Parts used Rhizome, leaf

Actions Circulatory stimulant, carminative, digestive, expectorant, diuretic, antiemetic, analgesic, anti-inflammatory, diaphoretic, antispasmodic, immune tonic, antimicrobial, antioxidant.

Digestion Warming digestive stimulant; improves appetite and digestion. Useful in anorexia. • Removes accumulation of toxins, enhancing immunity. • Relieves pain and spasm, indigestion, distension and wind, nausea, IBS and food allergies. • Relieves griping from diarrhoea, travel and morning sickness and hangovers.

Circulation Stimulates the heart and circulation, and reduces blood clotting; used for poor peripheral circulation, chilblains and Raynaud's disease.

Respiratory system Antispasmodic and expectorant; relieves asthma, catarrhal coughs, chest infections, bronchitis and bronchietasis. • Hot tea taken at the onset of sore throat, cold or flu brings down fevers, clears catarrh and helps resolve infection.

Immune system Volatile oils dispel acute bacterial and viral infections such as colds, flu, bronchitis, bacterial dysentery and malaria. Used in East for epidemics such as cholera. • Anti-inflammatory and antioxidant; inhibits prostaglandin synthesis and aids immunity and circulation; used for osteo- and rheumatoid arthritis.

Reproductive system Promotes menstruation; used for delayed/scanty periods and clots. • Relieves spasm, pain at ovulation and menstruation and in endometriosis. • Ancient reputation as an aphrodisiac. Its invigorating properties are helpful for impotence.

CAUTION Avoid with peptic ulcers and gallstones.

Drug interactions Avoid with anticoagulants.

PART III:
COMMON AILMENTS

The most common health conditions
that respond to herbal remedies are
profiled in this chapter. The ailments
are organized by body system, and
each treatment protocol offers advice
on herbs to be used and effective
methods of their administration.
Supportive action is suggested for
each condition, including changes to
diet and lifestyle and supplements
that could augment herbal treatment.
Brief case studies illustrate the
effectiveness of these treatments.

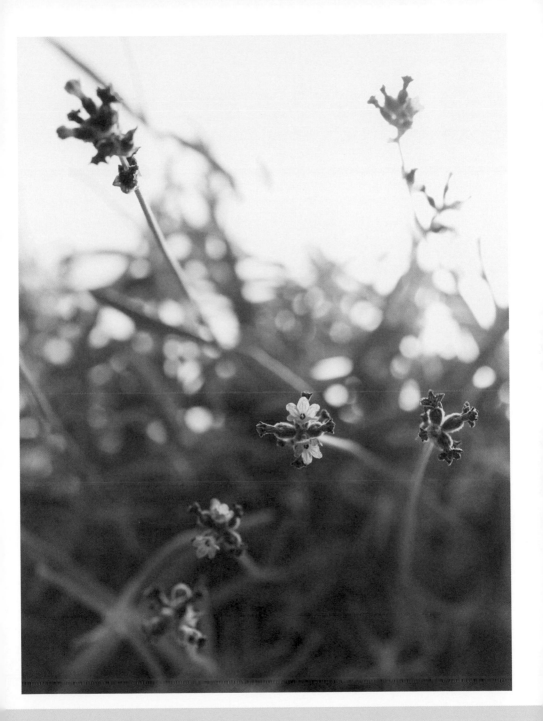

HERBS AND THE NERVOUS SYSTEM

There are many wonderfully beneficial herbs that have a direct effect on the nervous system and the world of herbs offers a range of therapeutic strategies for dealing with a number of specific nervous problems. There are herbs to lift the spirits, calm anxiety, relax muscles, increase memory and concentration and aid sleep. There are other herbs, known as adaptogens, that have an impressive ability to improve energy and vitality and enhance a person's resilience to stress.

TENSION AND ANXIETY

Tension or anxiety is a normal response to a difficult situation, which should settle once the problem is resolved. It can become habitual when we are run-down either by long-term stress, nutritional deficiencies, excess alcohol and caffeine, or lack of exercise and sleep.

Treatment

Effective calming herbs for acute anxiety include Passion flower, Wild lettuce and Wild oats taken every hour or two hours if necessary. Chamomile or Lemon balm tea is also soothing. For chronic problems, adaptogens like Ginseng, Ashwagandha, Bacopa, Polygonum, Schisandra, Shatavari, Bhringaraj, Liquorice and Holy basil will strengthen the nerves. Other good anxiolytic herbs include Vervain, St John's wort, California poppy, Rose, Motherwort, Lime flower, Hops, Lavender, Rosemary and Peony.

Also very effective are hot herbal baths and massage using relaxing essentials oils of Holy basil, Nutmeg, Lavender, Rosemary, Rose or Chamomile. A few drops of any of these in a base of sesame oil will ease muscle tension and soothe anxiety.

Other measures

For patients suffering from tension and anxiety, regular aerobic exercise is often advised alongside any herbal treatments. This will stimulate endorphins and increase resilience. Meditation cultivates calmness and a sense of control, Pranayama (breathing exercises) is calming, and inhalations of Frankincense oil deepen breathing. Patients should avoid caffeine, sugar, alcohol and any unnecessary drugs, which can reduce resistance to stress.

DEPRESSION

Treatment
Mood-elevating Wild oats, Vervain, St John's wort and Siberian ginseng taken three times daily can appreciably lift the spirits and replace essential nutrients necessary for the nervous system. Lemon balm, Borage, St John's wort, Wild oats, Holy basil and Wood betony taken three to six times daily can help acute depression. Adding essential oils of Lavender, Rosemary, Chamomile or Rose to baths and/or massage oils can also help.

Rosemary, Rhodiola, Gotu kola, Siberian ginseng, Liquorice and Wild oats are great adaptogens, excellent for debility and depression following illness or long-term stress. Rose, Shatavari, Chaste tree, Evening primrose, Black cohosh and St John's wort are appropriate for depression related to hormone imbalance

INSOMNIA

Treatment
For problems getting off to sleep, use Hops, Passion flower, Chamomile, Lemon balm, Lime flower, Wild oats, Wild lettuce or Valerian as teas, or 1–3 teaspoons of tincture before bed. A teaspoonful of Nutmeg is good taken in hot milk at bedtime. For problems staying asleep, try taking Ashwagandha, Bacopa, Wild oats, Hops, Passion flower, St John's wort or Valerian.

A warm sesame oil massage followed 10–15 minutes later by a bath before bed can work wonders. Add strong infusions/oils of Lavender, Chamomile, Neroli or Rose to the bath for added effect.

Other measures
Allowing 45 minutes of quiet time before retiring is important. It is best to avoid all caffeine and have regular meals, exercise and sleep times and no sleep during the day, to settle the nervous system.

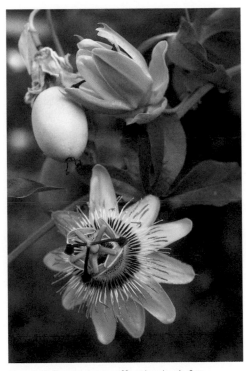

Passion flower is an effective herb for calming anxiety, relaxing tense muscles and promoting sleep.

HEADACHE AND MIGRAINE

These may be warning signs of stress or fatigue, or related to eyestrain, sinusitis, hormonal imbalances, allergy, liver and digestive problems, dysbiosis, pollution, poor diet, high blood pressure, low blood sugar, alcohol or back problems.

Treatment
Effective preventative herbs include Lemon balm, Rosemary, Feverfew, Wood betony, Bacopa and Gingko.

At the first signs of pain, take relaxant and painkilling herbs such as Passion flower, California poppy, Hops, Pasque flower, St John's wort, Wild lettuce, Rosemary, Chamomile or Vervain and repeat as necessary. You can also use anti-inflammatory herbs: Meadowsweet, Black willow, Ginger or Lavender. Inhale Lavender, Peppermint or Rosemary oils, or massage them into the temples.

Liver herbs Dandelion, Burdock, Vervain, Holy thistle and Milk thistle are important to detoxify the system. Chaste tree, Shatavari or Wild yam and Evening primrose oil will help address hormone imbalances. Massage of the head and neck with Gotu kola oil can bring relief.

Other measures
Avoid all caffeine and sugar as well as known migraine triggers – chocolate, cheese, alcohol and citrus fruits.

ADD AND ADHD

Attention deficit disorder (ADD) and attention deficit hyperactivity disorder (ADHD) have been linked to toxic metals, dysbiosis, food sensitivities, nutritional deficiencies and excess sugar. Impaired glucose metabolism may also be a major contributory factor, caused by excessive intake of simple carbohydrates and nutrient-poor junk foods. Lack of fresh air and exercise, hypoglycaemia and over-exposure to smoky atmospheres, noise, computers and television can all affect the brain adversely.

Treatment
Red clover, Pau d'arco, Coriander leaf, Bladderwrack and Nettle aid the elimination of heavy metals. These can be combined with cleansing herbs Milk thistle, Turmeric, Common grape vine, Barberry, Dandelion or Burdock to detoxify the system and protect against toxic damage. To aid sleep, use Ashwagandha, California poppy, Chamomile, Passion flower, Hops or Lime flower. Liquorice is helpful as an adrenal tonic.

Other measures
Avoiding allergenic foods including food colourings and additives, dairy produce, salicylates, wheat or gluten, corn, chocolate, caffeine, eggs and citrus fruits can be helpful. Supplements of B vitamins, magnesium and omega-3 essential fatty acids are recommended.

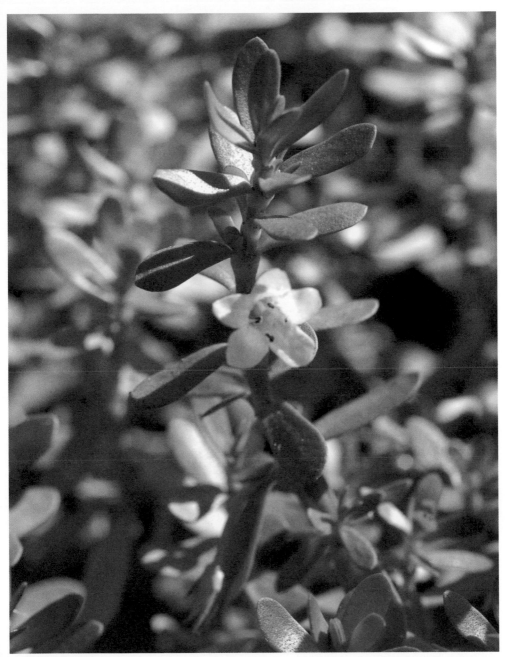

Bacopa is popular in India for boosting mental acuity, including concentration.

NEURALGIA AND SCIATICA

Inflammation or injury of a nerve can cause excruciating pain, as experienced by anyone who has suffered from sciatica, lumbago or trigeminal neuralgia. Nerves can be traumatized by injury, burns, cuts, slipped discs, vertebrae out of alignment, a tumour or muscle spasm. Heavy metals such as lead or mercury can damage nerves, as can alcoholism and diabetes.

To ensure recovery, the cause of the pain needs to be identified and treated. Where there is pressure on a nerve from a spinal problem, consult a chiropractor or osteopath.

Treatment

To relieve nerve pain, try California poppy, Hops, St John's wort, Wood betony, Pasque flower, Feverfew, Meadowsweet or Black cohosh, in acute doses if necessary. Cramp bark, Valerian, Passion flower, Lavender, Rosemary, Chamomile or Wild yam will help relax tense and painful muscles. Wild oats are wonderful 'nerve food' and help repair nerve tissue. Where circulation to the area is poor, Hawthorn, Cinnamon and Ginger will bring blood and nutrition to the area.

Externally, St John's wort oil, gently massaged into the area, is specific for damaged nerves and neuralgia, and is an excellent pain reliever. A few drops of Cayenne pepper tincture added to the oil will increase its pain-relieving properties. Start with one to two drops and gradually build up the ratio of Cayenne pepper, as it may have a tendency to cause a burning sensation in some people with hypersensitive nerves.

Other pain-relieving essential oils that can be used for massage in a base of sesame oil include Ginger, Rosemary, Lavender, Peppermint, Chamomile and Coriander.

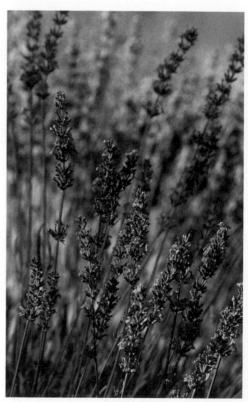

Lavender helps to reduce pain and has a soothing effect on the nervous system.

HERBS AND THE IMMUNE SYSTEM

The world of herbs is replete with immune stimulants that perform their work in a variety of ways. Some herbs increase the production and activity of macrophages – cells that the immune system sends to digest invaders – while others also stimulate the production of defence substances, such as interferon, which protect non-infected cells from viruses. Herbs can also enhance the production and function of T-cells – vital immune cells that kill viruses, fungi and certain bacteria. Immune-enhancing herbs include Ginseng, Guduchi, Cat's claw, Aswagandha, Liquorice, Echinacea, Olive leaf, Garlic, Shiitake and Reishi mushrooms and Turmeric.

FEVERS

A fever is the body's vital reaction to an infection and a symptom that the body is fighting invaders, whether they are bacterial, viral or fungal. Raising the internal thermostat enables the body to fight off the infection quickly, as it has a natural antibiotic and antiviral effect.

Treatment

At the first sign of fever it is best to fast in order to boost the immune system and drink plenty of fluids to aid elimination of toxins. If the patient is uncomfortable, he or she should take hot teas of diaphoretics like Chamomile, Lime flower or Meadowsweet every couple of hours to bring heat to the surface, cause sweating and hasten the elimination of heat and toxins.

Other good fever-reducing herbs include Willow bark, Vervain, Cleavers, Rose, Holy basil, Elderflower, Yarrow, Peppermint, Lavender and Lemon balm. Take singly, or in combinations every two hours and sponge the body with tepid infusions. Also take ½ teaspoon of either Echinacea, Andrographis, Pau d'arco, Neem, Myrrh or Cat's claw tincture every two hours to fight off infection.

Caution

Do not give herbs containing salicylates to children under 12 years of age.

INFECTIONS

There are many immune-enhancing herbs that strengthen and support our innate defence mechanisms and help prevent infection. Many have powerful antiviral and antibacterial effects should we succumb.

As prevention, add immune-enhancing spices, such as Ginger, Nutmeg, Coriander, Turmeric, Long pepper or Cinnamon to cooking daily, and drink Ginger tea before breakfast. Adaptogenic herbs such as Shiitake and Reishi mushrooms, Cat's claw, Guduchi, Bhringaraj, Ashwagandha, Shatavari and Ginseng are great preventatives.

Treatment

At first signs of infection, fast to boost immunity, drink plenty of fluids to aid the elimination of toxins and take ½ teaspoon of Echinacea, Wild indigo, Golden seal, Myrrh, Barberry, Andrographis or Pau d'arco tincture every two hours. Add a little Liquorice, which has antiviral and immune-enhancing properties.

Drink antimicrobial teas through the day: Dill, Marigold, Wild celery, Lemon balm, Chamomile, Lavender, Sage, Thyme, Rosemary or Rose.

Other measures

A healthy diet, good digestion (much of our immunity lies in the gut) and adequate exercise, rest and relaxation will support the immune system.

ALLERGIES

If a person's immune system reacts against substances that are not infectious or harmful, they have an allergy. Allergic symptoms include sneezing, runny or itchy nose, nasal congestion, itchy eyes, digestive disturbances, eczema and asthma. Stress, poor diet, nutritional deficiencies, pollution, drugs, injury, surgery, digestive problems, dysbiosis and genetic tendencies can all predispose to allergies.

Treatment

Treatment involves improving nutrition, temporarily avoiding the allergen and balancing digestive and immune systems. Adaptogenic herbs Ashwagandha, Guduchi, Amalaki, Liquorice, Shiitake and Reishi mushrooms, Shatavari, Aloe vera and Ginseng increase immunity and help prevent allergic reactions.

Cat's claw, Walnut, Burdock, Turmeric, Ginger, Myrrh, Cinnamon and Andrographis will combat dysbiosis, which predisposes to leaky gut syndrome and allergies. Chamomile, Nettle, Lemon balm and Yarrow soothe the allergic response and inhibit histamine, which is responsible for inflammatory symptoms.

Evening primrose oil or Borage seed oil will provide gamma-linolenic acid (GLA), deficiency of which is implicated in several allergic conditions.

Other measures

Minimize allergenic foods such as dairy produce, citrus fruits, chocolate, peanuts, wheat or gluten, shellfish, food colourings and preservatives. Avoid caffeine, alcohol, tobacco, sugar and junk foods, which increase susceptibility to allergies.

The severity of the inflammatory response can be diminished by vitamin C (500 mg twice daily) plus bioflavonoids and magnesium (500 mg daily), which are natural antihistamines. Quercetin, a bioflavonoid found in citrus fruits, helps to inhibit the secretion of histamine, leukotrienes and prostaglandins. Other flavonoid-containing foods and herbs could also prove helpful, as they have anti-inflammatory, antioxidant and immunoregulating properties. Capillary-strengthening magnesium with vitamins B and C has an antihistamine action1 and can be taken at the onset of symptoms.

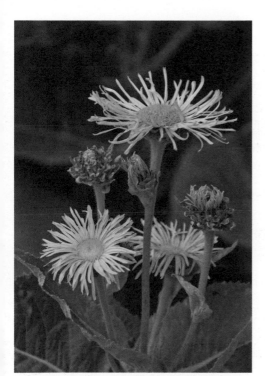

Elecampane is an excellent tonic for the respiratory system, combating infection and clearing congestion.

CHRONIC FATIGUE SYNDROME (CFS)

Also known as post-viral fatigue syndrome or ME (myalgic encephalomyelitis), CFS is common between the ages of 25 and 45, and is characterized by prolonged fatigue and other symptoms including poor memory and concentration, swollen glands, muscle/joint pain, headaches, poor sleep and malaise after exertion.

It tends to follow an acute viral infection when immunity has been compromised by toxicity, drugs or alcohol, poor diet, depression, dysbiosis or stress caused by a major life event like bereavement or job loss.

Treatment

Adaptogenic herbs Ashwagandha, Shatavari, Liquorice, Guduchi, Amalaki, Rehmannia, Shiitake and Reishi mushrooms, Rhodiola or

Siberian ginseng are excellent for increasing resistance to stress and strengthening immunity.

Ginkgo and Gotu kola enhance memory and concentration and relieve depression. St John's wort, Lemon balm and Vervain are effective antidepressants.

Black cohosh, Turmeric, Frankincense, Devil's claw and Ginger help alleviate joint and muscle pain.

Take a cup of Ginger tea before breakfast to improve digestion and

Andrographis, Cat's claw, Burdock, Neem, Myrrh and Olive leaf to combat dysbiosis.

Other measures

Eliminate inflammatory foods from the diet, including refined carbohydrates, saturated fats, alcohol and caffeine, and take vitamin supplements, coenzyme Q10, magnesium, B vitamins and zinc to support the immune system and increase energy. A supplement of bromelain from pineapple is recommended for easing joint and muscle pain.

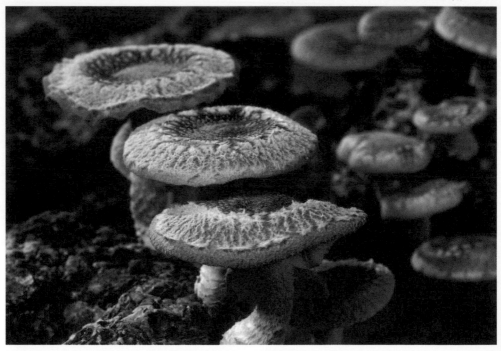

Shiitake mushrooms are adaptogens, enhancing immunity and increasing the body's ability to cope with stress.

HERBS AND THE RESPIRATORY SYSTEM

The herbal approach to the treatment of respiratory problems is firstly prevention through diet, lifestyle and herbs to maximize immunity and resistance to infections. Herbs such as Echinacea, Garlic, Thyme, Ginger and Turmeric all have effective immunostimulatory as well as antimicrobial actions.

COLDS AND FLU

The common cold virus can thrive only where the conditions in the body are right, and this is more likely to be the case when we are run-down, stressed, take insufficient exercise, have sluggish bowels, a poor diet, dysbiosis, or our bodies are overloaded with toxins. The resulting symptoms, particularly fevers and catarrh, are the body's way of clearing toxins.

Treatment

At the first signs of infection, take a hot infusion of Elderflower, Peppermint and Yarrow every one to two hours to relieve aches and pains, reduce fever and clear catarrh. Ginger tea or hot Lemon with honey is also excellent. At the same time take ½ teaspoon of Echinacea tincture and 500 mg of vitamin C every two hours. Other immune-enhancing, antimicrobial and decongestant spices, like Cinnamon, Cardamom, Fenugreek, Turmeric and Coriander, improve digestion and balance the gut flora and can be taken similarly. Andrographis, Elderberry and Elderflower, Garlic, Golden seal, Lemon balm, Pau d'arco, Cat's claw, Amalaki and Wormwood are other effective remedies to combat infection and reduce fevers.

Aromatic inhalations or hot foot baths of Rosemary, Lavender, Thyme, Cinnamon or Chamomile will all reduce swelling of mucous membranes and loosen and clear catarrh. A Ginger or Mustard foot bath can be effective, too.

Other measures

Supplements of vitamin C and zinc will help to prevent and decrease the duration of a cold.

CATARRH AND SINUSITIS

Irritation and inflammation of the nasal passages and sinuses from infection or inhaled pollutants causes extra secretion of mucus as a protective mechanism, which accumulates as catarrh. This can lead to sinusitis, which can be very painful and result in headaches and post-nasal drip, causing recurrent throat and chest problems. Chronic catarrh and sinusitis can be due to infection, environmental pollution, poor diet or food allergy, or a sign of intestinal dysbiosis and toxicity.

Treatment

Take antimicrobial herbs Golden seal, Wild indigo, Elderberry, Andrographis, Echinacea, Neem, Amalaki, Turmeric, Garlic or Myrrh to enhance immunity, combat infections in the respiratory system and clear toxicity from the gut. These are best combined with decongestants and astringents taken in hot teas, such as Ginger, Cinnamon, Coriander, Thyme, Ground ivy, Yarrow, Elderflower, Chamomile, Eyebright, Agrimony, Meadowsweet and Peppermint.

Demulcents like Slippery elm, Marshmallow, Mullein and Plantain soothe irritation and sinus pain.

Oils of Lavender, Peppermint, Rosemary, Thyme or Chamomile are good in inhalations and baths, or used for massage around the nose and sinuses.

Other measures

Washing the sinuses by sniffing salt water can work wonders. Omitting wheat or gluten, dairy produce and sugar from the diet and taking a supplement of vitamin C is recommended.

EARACHE

Earache can arise from pain and inflammation in the throat, tonsils, gums, teeth or parotid glands, or inflammation of the outer ear. Acute middle ear infection (otitis media) causes acute pain and is common in children. Children treated with antibiotics are prone to recurrent antibiotic-resistant strains of ear infection and glue ear. Other underlying causes include dysbiosis, passive smoking, chronic catarrh and throat, tonsil and sinus infection.

Treatment

For ear infections, use a combination of internal and local herbs. Chamomile is an excellent antimicrobial, anti-inflammatory and pain reliever for children. Echinacea enhances the immune system's fight against infection. Elderberry, Garlic, Golden seal, Andrographis, Wild indigo and Cat's claw are also good antimicrobials and will combat infection and reduce fevers.

Elderflower, Plantain, Thyme, Ground ivy and Meadowsweet help clear catarrh and alleviate pain. Pasque flower is specific for pain. Cleavers, Dandelion, Blue flag and Poke root help reduce swollen glands that can cause congestion in the middle ear.

Provided there is no pus from a perforated eardrum, you can drop warm Mullein, St John's wort or

Olive oil blended with a few drops of either Lavender, Garlic or Chamomile oil into the patient's ear and plug it with cotton wool to relieve inflammation or infection. Avoid including mucus-producing foods in the diet, such as sugar, junk foods and dairy produce.

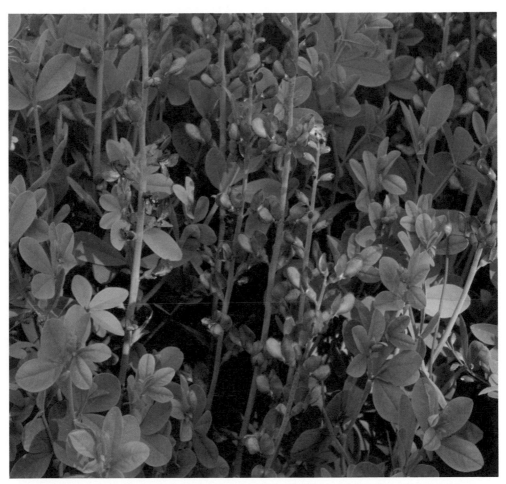

Wild indigo is an antimicrobial herb with antiseptic properties used to boost the body's immune system.

SORE THROAT AND SWOLLEN GLANDS

Generally a prelude to a bacterial or viral infection, sore throats can also be caused by irritation of the throat lining by tobacco smoke, post-nasal drip, allergies, acid reflux, dry heat and shouting. Swelling of lymph glands in the neck indicate that the body is attempting to fight off infection, or is overloaded with toxins and increasing the work of the lymphatic system in carrying away waste products.

Treatment

Antimicrobial herbs Echinacea, Wild indigo, Turmeric, Garlic, Wormwood, Cat's claw, Pau d'arco, Myrrh or Andrographis can be taken at the first signs to ward off infection.

Immune-enhancing Ashwagandha, Shatavari, Guduchi, Baikal Skullcap, Rehmannia, Shiitake and Reishi mushrooms, Schisandra and Amalaki help reduce allergies and inflammation caused by environmental irritants.

Demulcents Marshmallow, Slippery elm, Mullein, Aloe vera, Liquorice, Coltsfoot and Comfrey moisten and soothe irritation of the mucous membranes of the throat.

Cleavers, Poke root, Marigold, Blue flag, Burdock and Red clover enhance the lymphatic system in its cleansing and immune work.

Gargling or spraying the throat with Sage, Thyme, Sweet marjoram, Turmeric, Myrrh or salt water will also help.

Other measures

Supplements of vitamins A, B and C also enhance immunity.

Caution

If a child runs a fever with an acute sore throat and swollen tonsils, seek professional help. These symptoms could indicate a streptococcal infection with risk of further complications such as nephritis and rheumatic fever.

ASTHMA

This is caused by the release of inflammatory chemicals that inflame and narrow the bronchial tubes, making it difficult to breathe. Increased mucus production blocks the airways still further. Asthma can be triggered by food allergies, environmental pollutants, respiratory infections, immune problems (caused by suppression of eczema and chest infections for example), emotional problems, digestive disturbances or dysbiosis. Prevention is the best line of treatment. Herbs can be taken in conjunction with other medication or inhalants, and may need to be taken over several months. Treat the first signs of respiratory infection vigorously to prevent asthma from getting progressively worse.

Treatment

Expectorant herbs such as Elecampane, Thyme, Hyssop, Garlic, Coltsfoot, Ginger, Garlic, Liquorice and Mullein liquefy and clear mucus from the bronchial tubes, and strengthen and relax bronchial muscles, opening the airways.

Thyme, Elecampane, Pleurisy root, Angelica, Pau d'arco and Sweet marjoram are excellent for combating chest infections.

Adaptogens Schisandra, Ashwagandha, Shatavari, Liquorice, Turmeric or Shiitake and Reishi mushrooms enhance immunity, reduce inflammation and increase resilience to stress.

Ginkgo, Chamomile, Yarrow, Feverfew, Baikal Skullcap or Nettle help decrease allergic responses that may trigger asthma.

Relaxing herbs such as Holy basil, Rose, Lavender, Wild oats, Honeysuckle or Chamomile help reduce tension.

Caution

Seek medical attention in cases of acute asthma.

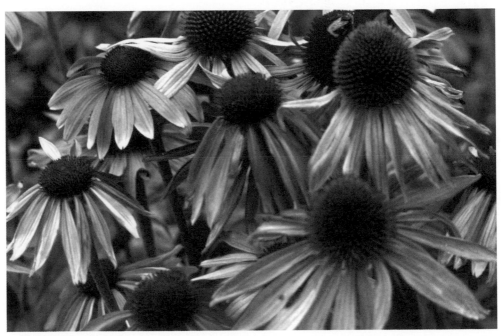

Echinachea, well-known as a herbal immune stimulant, is prescribed to prevent and treat all acute respiratory infections.

HAY FEVER

Hay fever, also known as allergic rhinitis, is a common atopic condition that mostly occurs when high concentrations of pollens are released during late spring and summer, especially during hot weather.

The familiar symptoms are caused by the release of histamine and other inflammatory chemicals, and are generally worse in the morning and evening, which coincides with the changes in air temperature. House dust and animal hair can also produce similar reactions. Hay fever as well as other atopic conditions like eczema and asthma tend to be genetic and occur when immunity is lowered, for example by long-term stress and dysbiosis.

Treatment

As a preventative, take immunostimulants Ashwagandha, Guduchi, Amalaki, Siberian ginseng or Echinacea and 1–2 dessertspoons of local honey in honeycombs with each meal for two to four months before the hay fever season.

Antihistamine and anti-inflammatory herbs Turmeric, Echinacea, Golden seal, Chamomile, Nettle, Lemon balm, Feverfew, Baikal skullcap or Yarrow with a little Liquorice help to reduce symptoms once they start and can be taken every 2 hours if necessary. They can also be used as teas for inhalations to ease symptoms.

Agrimony, Elderflower, Plantain and Eyebright tone mucous membranes and desensitize them to allergens. Marshmallow and Slippery elm soothe irritation of the mucosa.

Ginger, Garlic, Thyme, Burdock or Marigold combat dysbiosis, while Burdock, Dandelion, Agrimony and Milk thistle support the liver.

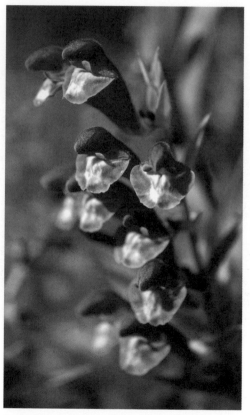

Baikal skullcap has antihistamine effects useful in the treatment of hay fever.

Other measures

Supplements of vitamin C and magnesium are recommended. Cutting out wheat or gluten and dairy foods is also helpful. Sunglasses may help to reduce eye irritation.

COUGHS AND BRONCHITIS

A cough is a reflex response designed to remove irritants such as dust, toxins, micro-organisms or mucus blocking the throat or bronchial tubes, but it can become chronic and debilitating, disturbing sleep. Coughs can be aggravated by both stress and cold weather.

Treatment

Demulcent herbs like Marshmallow, Mullein, Plantain, Liquorice, Coltsfoot or Slippery elm soothe irritation and inflammation in dry, tickly coughs.

Expectorants and decongestants including Thyme, Elecampane, Ground ivy, White horehound, Hyssop, Ginger, Angelica and Sweet marjoram liquefy and clear phlegm. Vitamin C in Elderberries and Blueberries/ Bilberries, as well as infusions of Rose petals, stimulate the mucociliary escalator, clear phlegm and protect the lungs from infection.

Nervous coughs can be eased with relaxing herbs such as Chamomile, Lemon balm and Holy basil. Antimicrobials including Thyme, Elecampane, Hyssop, Cat's claw, Pau

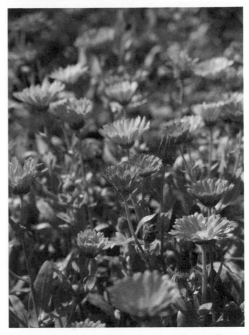

Marigold can help soothe irritated eyes for sufferers of hay fever.

d'arco, Garlic, Cinnamon and Pleurisy root combat infection and support the immune system. A cough formula will need to consist of mixtures of these herbs, depending on the nature of the cough.

Essential oils of Rosemary, Rose, Thyme, Ginger or Cinnamon can be used in baths and inhalation.

Caution

Fever and malaise with cough, green phlegm or breathlessness may indicate acute bronchitis or pneumonia. Seek medical attention if any of these symptoms present.

HERBS AND THE DIGESTIVE SYSTEM

The herbal materia medica offers a huge range of remedies for almost every kind of digestive disorder. For example, warming spices such as Ginger, Cinnamon and Long pepper will stimulate the secretion of digestive enzymes; mucilage-rich herbs including Slippery elm and Marshmallow soothe irritation; Fennel, Peppermint and Chamomile ease pain and spasm, and bitter herbs such as Dandelion, Agrimony and Burdock support the liver.

CONSTIPATION

It is important to ascertain and treat the causes of constipation and not become reliant on laxative medicines, which can be taken short term but may aggravate the problem in the long run. Causes include lack of exercise, ignoring the urge, old age, piles, IBS, diverticulitis, food allergy, dysbiosis, nutritional deficiency, excess refined foods, insufficient fibre from fruit, vegetables and whole grains, and tension in the bowel due to stress. It is important to remedy constipation otherwise toxins from reabsorption in the bowel may cause chronic disease.

Treatment
Use Linseed, Fenugreek or Psyllium seeds to bulk out bowel contents and push them along. Soak 1–2 teaspoons of seeds in a cup of hot water for 2 hours, add lemon and honey if you like and drink at bedtime.

It is important to drink plenty of water. Liquorice, Dandelion root and Burdock root taken as decoctions 3 times a day are also effective for mild constipation. If necessary, add more stimulating laxative herbs such as Yellow dock or Senna pods with a little Ginger for a week or two.

For stress-related constipation, add Chamomile, Lemon balm, Dill, Hops or Cramp bark. Garlic, Thyme, Burdock or Marigold work well for dysbiosis.

Other measures
Live yogurt, lacto-acidophilus or Grapefruit seed extract can also help candida, which can predispose to constipation. Taking 30 minutes of exercise daily is recommended.

Caution
If constipation is persistent, develops suddenly or with pain, be sure to seek medical attention.

DIARRHOEA

Diarrhoea represents the body's attempt to rid itself of poisons or irritants (including drugs, chemicals and allergens), inflammation or infection in the gut, so it is important not to stop it but to address the underlying causes. It is vital to drink plenty of fluids to replace lost water and electrolytes.

Treatment

Use astringent herbs such as Agrimony, Bayberry, Cinnamon, Raspberry leaf or Yarrow to dry up secretions and tone the gut. Demulcent herbs Slippery elm and Marshmallow soothe irritation and act as prebiotics to support beneficial flora in the gut.

Chamomile, Hops, Wild yam, Dill and Lemon balm reduce anxiety in stress-related diarrhoea. Digestives Ginger, Cinnamon, Turmeric and Coriander, taken regularly as teas or in food, enhance the secretion of digestive enzymes.

For infection causing gastroenteritis and dysbiosis, use antimicrobials including Golden seal, Thyme, Chamomile, Cinnamon, Pau d'arco, Garlic and Ginger.

Antispasmodics such as Peppermint, Ginger, Dill and Chamomile relieve cramping pain and Chamomile, Hops, Golden seal, Meadowsweet and Yarrow relieve inflammation.

Other measures

Wheat or gluten and dairy foods can cause food intolerances, while red meat and too much hard, raw food can be indigestible and aggravate the condition, so these are best avoided until fully recovered. Acidophilus supplements are also useful.

Caution

If diarrhoea persists or is accompanied by fever, or if there is mucus or blood in stools, seek medical attention.

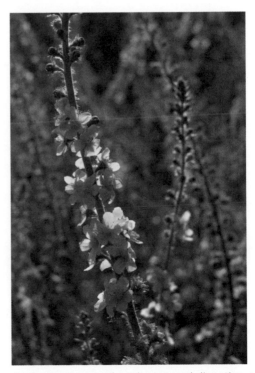

Agrimony is a good astringent and digestive tonic and can be helpful in relieving diarrhoea.

IRRITABLE BOWEL SYNDROME (IBS)

The bowel can become irritated by poorly digested and putrefying foods caused by weak digestion, stress, poor diet and disturbance of gut flora by, for example, antibiotics. Accumulated toxins, loss of beneficial flora and increase of pathogenic organisms cause dysbiosis, which leads to leaky gut syndrome, food intolerances and lowered immunity. Resulting symptoms include alternating diarrhoea and constipation, flatulence and abdominal discomfort.

Treatment

Anti-inflammatory and antispasmodic herbs such as Chamomile, Wild yam, Cramp bark, Meadowsweet, Peppermint, Hops or Myrrh can be helpful. Demulcents like Slippery elm, Aloe vera and Marshmallow are soothing and healing, while astringent Yarrow, Thyme, Agrimony and Bayberry protect the gut wall from irritation. Relaxants such as Lemon balm, Vervain, Dill, Hops or Valerian can help reduce stress. Bilberries are helpful for diarrhoea and Burdock can be taken for constipation.

To address dysbiosis and enhance immunity, Cat's claw, Chamomile, Cinnamon, Golden seal, Echinacea, Myrrh, Amalaki, Aloe vera, Olive leaf, Common grape vine, Garlic or Turmeric are recommended. Drinking Ginger tea before meals and adding mild spices to cooking will stimulate the secretion of digestive enzymes and help maintain healthy gut flora.

Other measures

Food intolerance is implicated in many cases, so temporarily omit tea, coffee, dairy products, eggs and wheat or gluten from your diet.

Caution

Consult your doctor if there is mucus or blood in stools or severe abdominal pain.

INFLAMMATORY BOWEL DISEASE (IBD)

Chronic inflammation of the gut is a serious problem that can involve ulceration and bleeding that sometimes necessitates surgery. It is indicated by severe abdominal pain, nausea, diarrhoea or constipation, blood in the stools, poor appetite, weight loss, fever as well as lethargy. The most common forms of IBD are autoimmune problems such as ulcerative colitis and Crohn's disease, which can be sparked off by an bacterial or viral infection and may cause poor absorption and nutritional deficiencies that in turn lead to anaemia and osteoporosis.

Treatment

Turmeric and Frankincense are wonderful anti-inflammatory herbs and can be very effective for reducing pain and inflammation.

Chamomile tea taken frequently through the day is excellent. Liquorice, Cat's claw, Golden seal, Myrrh, Hops, Peppermint, Yarrow, Meadowsweet and Sarsaparilla are also helpful.

Ground Flax seed in water or Flax oil, Aloe vera juice, Marshmallow and Slippery elm soothe the gut lining and help regulate the bowels.

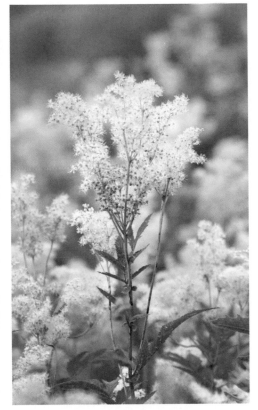

Meadowsweet reduces acidity in the stomach and has an anti-inflammatory action on the intestines.

Lemon balm, Hops, Chamomile, Wild oats, Ashwagandha and Passion flower are all recommended for reducing tension and anxiety.

Other measures
Avoid possible food allergens, particularly wheat or gluten and dairy products, as well as acidic and spicy foods, citrus fruits, tomatoes, alcohol and coffee. Bromelain from pineapple and papain from papaya help resolve inflammation and speed healing. Also, try to avoid getting tired and stressed, as this can aggravate IBD symptoms.

Caution
Seek medical attention if there is blood in the stool, a change in bowel habits lasting longer than 10 days or any of the above symptoms that do not improve with treatment.

NAUSEA AND VOMITING

Nausea and vomiting may result from adverse reactions to foods or drugs, nervous tension, migraine or infections causing irritation and inflammation in the stomach. Other causes include early weeks of pregnancy, travel sickness, peptic ulcers, gastritis, shock, intestinal obstruction, pressure on the brain by fluid in altitude sickness or a tumour, or loss of balance caused by inner ear infection. When symptoms present, it is important to drink plenty of fluid to prevent dehydration.

Treatment

The best and most delicious remedy for nausea and vomiting is fresh Ginger, sipped in tea or simply chewed. This is particularly useful in pregnancy when other herbs might be contraindicated. Teas of Chamomile, Fennel or Peppermint can also settle the stomach.

If symptoms are caused by emotional stress, teas or tinctures of Lemon balm, Chamomile, Lavender, Hops, Dill or Passion flower can help.

For an infection or food poisoning, take Garlic, Turmeric, Chamomile, Echinacea, Cinnamon, Pau d'arco or Golden seal every two hours.

Feverfew, Wood betony or Rosemary are best used when there are headaches or migraine, while Marshmallow and Slippery elm will soothe irritation, and Meadowsweet, Gentian and Burdock can reduce heat and inflammation in the stomach.

Caution

If symptoms persist or there is severe vomiting with high fever, seek medical attention.

HEARTBURN AND ACIDITY

These indicate a disordered stomach, hyperacidity and gastro-oesophageal reflux, which can be caused by chronic constipation, obesity or stress. They can also be triggered by alcohol, chocolate, sugar, refined carbohydrates, tea, coffee, cigarettes, rich, fatty, spicy and acidic foods such as tomatoes and citrus fruits, emotional upset and eating too fast. Heartburn and acidity can be aggravated by bending over, sitting hunched up and lying in bed.

Treatment

Try sipping Chamomile tea frequently. Meadowsweet is also cooling and soothing. Surprisingly, some people find that chewing fresh Ginger can ease their feelings of discomfort.

Demulcent herbs such as Marshmallow or Liquorice can soothe pain and reduce acidity. A gruel made with 1–2 teaspoons of Slippery elm powder mixed with warm water can bring almost instant relief. Taking 25 ml (1 fl oz) Aloe vera juice twice daily can also be effective, cooling heat and inflammation and combating symptoms caused by dysbiosis.

Peppermint, Lemon balm, Holy basil and Dill are excellent digestives and reduce tension in the gut, while bitter herbs like Dandelion root and Burdock are gently laxative, enhance digestion and reduce heat and burning. Chamomile, Hops, Vervain or Lemon balm are good when heartburn is related to stress.

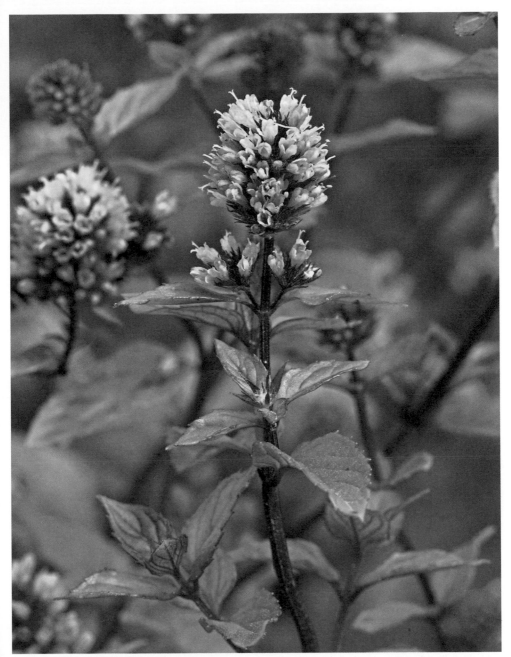

Peppermint soothes and relaxes the digestive system, and reduces bloating and wind.

LIVER PROBLEMS

The liver is the largest and perhaps most overworked organ in the human body and performs many vital functions, including filtering and breaking down toxins from the blood, making amino acids for protein production, metabolizing carbohydrates, protein and fats, storing nutrients absorbed from the gut, producing cholesterol and bile, and manufacturing urea. Liver disease is mainly caused by drinking excess alcohol, hepatitis, autoimmune diseases, poisons or drugs, and inherited disorders. Less serious, but widespread, is poor liver function, which causes a wide range of metabolic and hormonal problems, poor immune function, skin problems and allergies.

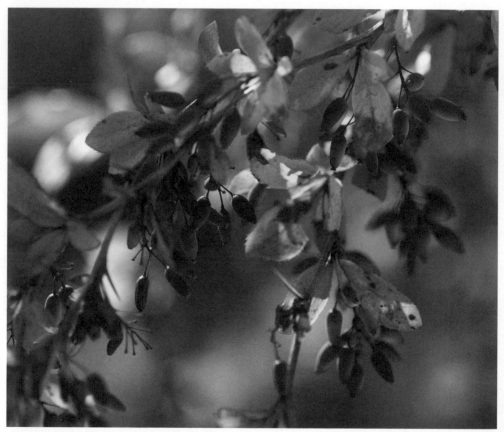

Barberry stimulates the liver to secrete bile and the gall bladder to regulate its flow, helpful in treating problems in these organs.

Treatment

Cholagogues are bitters such as Barberry, Yellow dock, Oregon grape, Rosemary, Vervain, Wormwood, Burdock, Dandelion and Guduchi, and can be taken to stimulate the flow of bile and support the liver in its work.

Barberry, Golden seal, Turmeric, Milk thistle, Marigold, Liquorice, Bhringaraj, Neem, Amalaki and St John's wort are antivirals that can be used for acute liver infections.

Some amazing adaptogenic herbs, including Guduchi, Andrographis, Neem, Milk thistle, Schisandra, Globe artichoke, Shiitake and Reishi mushrooms, Sarsaparilla and Rehmannia, protect the liver from damage from drugs and toxic chemicals.

Other measures

It is important to avoid alcohol, unnecessary drugs, caffeine and junk foods.

PARASITES

Most people have some kind of intestinal parasite, such as threadworms, roundworms or tapeworms, or protozoa such as amoeba and giardia. Their presence increases allergic tendencies, bleeding, loss of nutrients, bowel disturbances, aches and pains, and even migraine. Parasites spread easily, often via pets. Their eggs may be ingested with vegetables or fruit, or by putting contaminated fingers in the mouth. If someone has worms, treat the whole family and pets too.

Treatment

Anthelmintic herbs eliminate parasites and need to be taken for one to two weeks. Take one to two Garlic cloves, finely chopped, in 1 teaspoon of honey or warm milk 30 minutes before breakfast. Olive leaf, Pau d'arco, Bhringaraj, Andrographis, Neem, Myrrh, Wormwood, Barberry, Marigold, Gotu kola, Ginger, Wild carrot, Holy basil, Elecampane or Walnut are also effective taken on an empty stomach. Add laxatives Liquorice, Yellow dock or Dandelion root to speed the expulsion of worms.

Apply oil of Lavender, Neem, Rosemary or Thyme in ointment to the anus at night to prevent worms from laying eggs and relieve itching.

Horseradish, Long pepper and Cayenne pepper are all toxic to worms and can be added to food, along with pumpkin seeds, raw onion, grated carrot and carrot juice.

Check the stools daily for worms and repeat treatment after 2 weeks.

Other measures

It is best to avoid all sugary foods and refined carbohydrates in the diet, and to make sure that you eat live yogurt daily.

HERBS AND THE URINARY SYSTEM

Many herbs that exert their action on the urinary system can be used preventatively and therapeutically. Mucilaginous herbs such as Marshmallow, Corn silk, Comfrey leaf and Wild oats soothe irritation and inflammation. Aromatic herbs rich in antimicrobial volatile oils with a diuretic action, including Chamomile, Fennel, Lemon balm, Thyme and Coriander, taken regularly as teas or in food are excellent for helping to prevent infection. Cranberry and Blueberry/Bilberry are also valuable, helping to prevent infection by preventing pathogenic bacteria from sticking to the walls of the urinary tract. During any kind of infection or inflammatory process, diuretic herbs to increase the flow of urine such as Wild celery seed, Cleavers, Dandelion leaf, Corn silk, Couch grass and Bearberry can help the body to throw off accumulated toxins and debris produced as a result of the immune system's fight against infection and inflammation.

URINARY TRACT INFECTIONS

Infections tend to affect women more than men due to anatomical differences, but in men they can be caused by prostate problems. Cystitis refers to unpleasant urinary symptoms caused by irritation as well as infection, which are mostly from E. coli bacteria. Underlying causes include lowered immunity, dysbiosis, nutritional deficiencies, insufficient fluids, stress, excess alcohol/caffeine, blood sugar problems and sex.

Treatment
Antiseptic diuretics Buchu, Bearberry, Golden seal, Goldenrod, Chamomile, Fennel, Coriander, Sarsaparilla or Yarrow help combat infection and flush out bacteria, debris and irritants. Soothing Marshmallow, Plantain, Slippery elm, Comfrey leaf, Corn silk and Couch grass relieve irritation, pain and inflammation. Horsetail is soothing and healing, particularly useful for repairing damage after repeated infection. For irritation causing incontinence or bed-wetting, use Marshmallow, Bayberry, Horsetail, Gravel root or Yarrow. Drink lukewarm-to-cool teas of any of these every one to two hours in acute infections and three times daily in chronic problems. To relieve the burning/passing-broken-glass sensation, sit in a bath of strong Chamomile tea for 10–15 minutes.

Blueberries/Bilberries prevent bacteria from sticking to the walls of the urinary tract and are excellent as a preventative. Soups and juices made from Carrots, Parsley, Asparagus, Celery, Leeks and Garlic are also helpful.

Other measures

To prevent infection and irritation, drink 3–4 litres (5¼–7 pints) fluid daily to flush toxins and bacteria out of the body. During infection, drink plenty of water, herb teas or soothing barley water throughout the day.

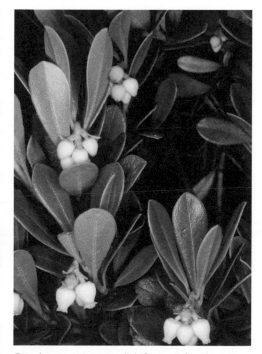

Bearberry acts as a disinfectant for the urinary system, thanks to its natural antibacterial properties.

FLUID RETENTION

Excess water in the tissues causes oedema, cellulite, swelling and discomfort, particularly in the feet and legs, where fluid accumulates first (due to gravity). It can occur temporarily in women premenstrually and during pregnancy, hot weather and long flights. More chronic fluid retention can be caused by thyroid problems, obesity, poor circulation, varicose veins and poor diet, especially insufficient protein. Oedema can indicate kidney and heart problems, which require professional treatment.

Treatment

Diuretics including Dandelion leaf, Wild celery seed, Nettle, Cleavers, Fennel, Coriander, Buchu, Meadowsweet, Corn silk, Chamomile and Bearberry aid the elimination of water through the kidneys and help reduce fluid retention. Add Chaste tree and Lady's mantle for premenstrual problems, including tender, swollen breasts.

Yarrow, Gingko, Gotu kola, Golden seal, Garlic, Lime flower and Hawthorn improve venous circulation and relieve swelling and discomfort in the legs and ankles. Antioxidants such as Blueberry/Bilberry, Elderberry and Horse chestnut strengthen and heal blood vessels. Bladderwrack and Guggulu are both helpful for treating low thyroid function and aiding weight reduction.

Other measures:

Excess sodium in salty foods increases fluid retention, so should be avoided, while potassium in foods like bananas, tomatoes and green vegetables encourages the elimination of sodium. It is important to take plenty of exercise, to raise the feet when sitting and avoid tea, coffee and alcohol. For premenstrual problems, take supplements of B-complex vitamins.

KIDNEY STONES

Infection and irritation in the kidney and insufficient fluids can lead to the formation of crystals, which develop into stones and gravel. They are mostly formed from calcium oxalate, calcium phosphate and uric acid. When they move they cause sudden, pain, which passes once the stones have passed out of the bladder.

Treatment

Use antilithic and diuretic herbs including Wild carrot, Gravel root, Blueberry/Bilberry, Buchu, Dandelion leaves, Goldenrod or Bearberry to dissolve and facilitate the passing of stones and gravel. These also combat urinary tract infection.

Demulcent diuretics Marshmallow, Comfrey leaf, Corn silk and Couch grass reduce inflammation, soothe and heal irritated urinary tubules, dissolve stones and gravel and ease their passing.

Antispasmodics Chamomile, Cramp bark, Wild yam, Passion flower and Valerian can help reduce pain and muscle spasm in the urinary tract caused by passing stones.

Other measures

Plenty of fluids and foods rich in magnesium and B vitamins help reduce the formation of stones.

PROSTATE PROBLEMS

The prostate is a walnut-sized gland surrounding the urethra, which carries urine from the bladder to the penis. An enlarged or swollen prostate obstructs the flow of

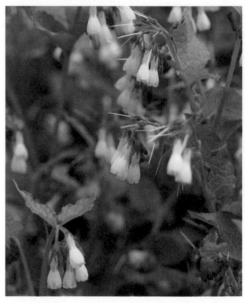

Comfrey leaf is one of several herbs that can dissolve kidney stones.

urine and causes sensations of pressure, hesitancy or urgency to empty the bladder. Incomplete bladder emptying predisposes to urinary infections and disturbs sleep through frequent trips to the toilet. Benign prostatic hypertrophy (BPH) commonly affects men from their late 40s and is related to dwindling testosterone levels and conversion of testosterone into dihydrotestosterone (DHT), which is linked to deficiencies of zinc, vitamin B6 and essential fatty acids. Infection (prostatitis) and cancer can also cause enlargement of the prostate.

Treatment

The best herb for shrinking the prostate is Saw palmetto when taken long term. Liquorice prevents conversion of testosterone to DHT and so prevents enlargement. Other useful herbs include Golden seal, Nettle root, Red clover, Horsetail, Dandelion, Gravel root, Siberian ginseng, Red grape seed extract, Evening primrose oil or Borage seed oil, Chinese angelica, Echinacea or Goldenrod.

For prostatitis, use Nettle root, Echinacea, Golden seal, Garlic, Buchu, Bearberry, Chamomile or Couch grass, in acute doses if necessary, and drink Cranberry or Blueberry/Bilberry juice and plenty of water.

For cramping pain caused by infection or inflammation, use Cramp bark, Chamomile or Chinese angelica.

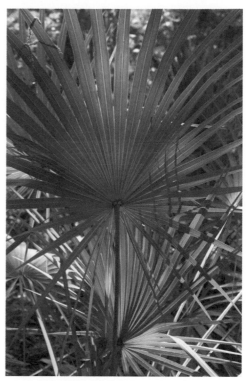

Saw palmetto is traditionally thought of as a man's herb and is prescribed to reduce enlarged prostate glands.

Other measures

A high-protein diet helps to maintain good testosterone levels. Increase zinc and essential fatty acid intake by eating pumpkin seeds daily and cooked tomatoes, which are rich in lycopene, as well as taking supplements of vitamins A, C and E, selenium and zinc.

Caution

If you suspect prostate problems, you should seek medical attention.

HERBS AND THE CIRCULATORY SYSTEM

Fruit, vegetables and herbs, including Blueberry/ Bilberry and Ginkgo, that are rich in antioxidants protect arteries from oxidation and reduce plaque deposits, while several other herbs, such as Lime flower, Gotu kola and Hawthorn, have the ability to regulate blood pressure, nourish the heart and strengthen the arteries. Fibres in complex carbohydrates such as Wild oats carry cholesterol out of cells, tissues and arteries to the liver, where it is excreted. Limiting salt and sugar intake, taking regular aerobic exercise and maintaining ideal body weight are also good preventative measures against circulatory disorders.

ANAEMIA

Lack of dietary iron, excess loss of blood (from heavy periods, haemorrhoids, bleeding gums or peptic ulcers) and those digestive problems that result in iron deficiency are the most common causes of anaemia. Vitamin B12 or folic acid deficiency can also cause anaemia, while other more serious problems, such as leukaemia or radiation therapy, can result in disturbance to red blood cells.

Treatment
Ashwagandha, Dandelion leaves, Blueberry/Bilberry, Raspberry leaves, Nettle, Yellow dock root, Codonopsis, Amalaki, Guggulu and Coriander leaves are all rich in iron and folic acid. Chinese angelica is rich in both vitamin B12 and folic acid, and increases red blood cell production.

To improve iron absorption, take iron-rich digestive herbs like Burdock, Vervain, Hawthorn, Gentian or Hops. Drinking a hot cup of tea made from fresh Ginger before meals will also aid iron absorption. Siberian ginseng increases resilience and strength in anaemia.

Other measures
Eat plenty of vitamin C-rich foods such as red, yellow and green vegetables and dark red fruit such as Blueberries/Bilberries, blackberries and blackcurrants, to enhance iron absorption. Avoid tea, coffee and alcohol, as they can inhibit iron absorption. Make sure that your diet is rich in iron, folic acid, protein and vitamins E and B12.

HEART CONDITIONS

There is much that can be done to prevent and heal heart problems, including dietary changes, exercise, nutritional supplements and herbs. Antioxidant herbs Turmeric, Blueberry/Bilberry, Hawthorn, Shiitake and Reishi mushrooms and Ginkgo can reduce oxidative damage to the heart and blood vessels caused by free radicals and strengthen the heart muscle by improving blood flow through the coronary arteries.

Treatment

Many herbs, such as Guggulu, Olive leaf, Hawthorn, Cayenne pepper, Red grape seed extract, Ginger, Turmeric, Evening primrose, Chinese angelica and Garlic can significantly lower blood pressure and low-density lipoprotein (LDL) cholesterol and prevent, and even reverse,

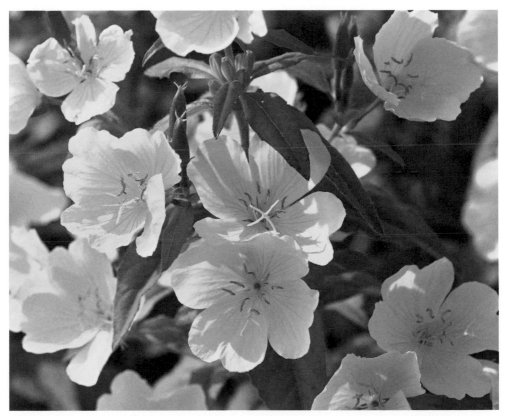

Evening primrose is prescribed to help lower blood pressure and keep platelets from clumping in the blood vessels.

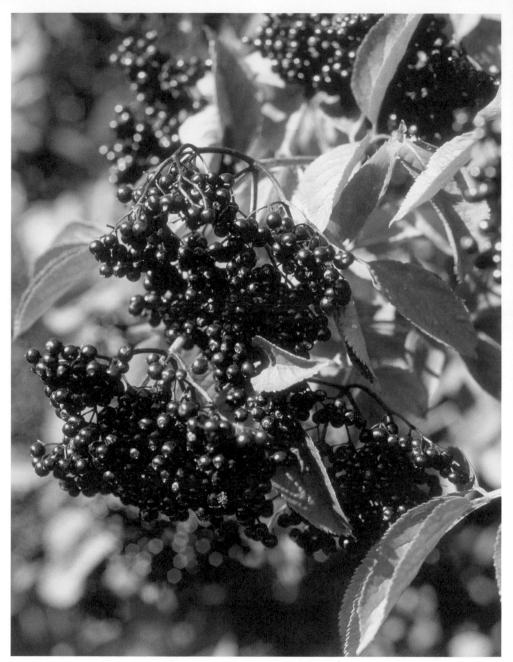

Elderberries are rich in flavonoids and oxidants and tone the walls of the small blood vessels.

atherosclerotic plaque from forming, thereby reducing the tendency to heart attacks.

Forskohlii relaxes the arteries, lowers blood pressure and improves blood flow through the heart, and is indicated in congestive heart failure, arteriosclerosis and angina. Angelica is a calcium-channel blocker in the heart, useful for high blood pressure, angina and heart arrhythmias. Astragalus is a good antioxidant and diuretic, and lowers blood pressure. It improves blood flow through the heart and heart function, and reduces ischaemic heart disease and angina.

Hawthorn, Motherwort, Lime flower, Lemon balm, Passion flower and Rosemary steady heart contractions and reduce palpitations. When these are related to menopausal flushes, add Sage or Black cohosh.

Other measures
Reduce or stop all caffeine intake such as coffee, cola and tea.

Caution
If you are on medication for a heart condition, check with your practitioner before taking herbs.

POOR CIRCULATION

Poor circulation to the extremities causes cold hands and feet and increases the tendency to chilblains and cramp. Chilblains are itchy, sore red lumps on fingers or toes that develop due to insufficient oxygen and nutrients being carried to the area by the blood. Poor circulation is caused by constriction of the arteries and can be inherited. It is aggravated by lack of exercise, smoking, caffeine, poor diet, tiredness and stress. Raynaud's syndrome and circulatory problems associated with heart or arterial disease can also cause circulatory problems.

Treatment
Circulatory stimulants include Ginger, Garlic, Cayenne pepper, Gotu kola, Coriander, Cinnamon, Prickly ash and Hawthorn. Hot teas of Yarrow, Peppermint, Elderflower, Rosemary and Lime flower increase blood flow, dilate arteries and reduce cramp. Blueberry/Bilberry and Horse chestnut improve circulation and strengthen blood vessels. Evening primrose and Borage seed oil also improve circulation.

Warm baths, foot baths or a massage using oils of Ginger, Cinnamon, Coriander, Sweet marjoram, Thyme or Rosemary are all good ways to relax tense muscles and stimulate blood flow. Marigold cream and Gotu kola and Lavender oil are useful for soothing chilblains.

Other measures
Supplements of vitamin C and bioflavonoids, omega-3 fatty acids and regular exercise are recommended.

CRAMP

Cramp is caused by muscular spasm and it can be very painful. Pregnant women and the elderly are more likely to suffer from cramp, and it may be a sign of low calcium levels, deficiencies of vitamins B or D, low digestive enzymes, poor absorption or circulatory problems.

Varicose veins, tiredness, lack of exercise, insufficient fluids and nervous tension may also be contributory factors.

Treatment
Effective circulatory stimulants include Ginger, Garlic, Gotu kola, Turmeric, Gingko, Hawthorn, Prickly ash, Cinnamon and Cayenne pepper. Amalaki, Guggulu and Coriander are also helpful. Hot teas of Ginger, Cinnamon, Cardamom, Yarrow, Peppermint and Elderflower also promote circulation and prevent cramp. Gotu kola, Blueberry/Bilberry and Gingko will aid venous return if there are varicose veins.

For cramps related to stress, tension and tiredness, use Cramp bark, Passion flower, Rosemary, Gotu kola, Holy basil, Lime flower or Ashwagandha.

Nettle, Dill, Wild oats, Wild celery seed, Borage, Meadowsweet, Dandelion leaves and Buchu are all rich in calcium and can be taken regularly as teas.

Massage with essential oils of Ginger, Cinnamon, Rosemary, Thyme or Sweet marjoram in a base of sesame oil to swiftly relieve pain.

Other measures
Moving the affected limb briskly, and walking and stretching are advisable. Take supplements of vitamin B and C, calcium and magnesium to support the nervous system and aid circulation.

HIGH BLOOD PRESSURE

An increase in pressure inside narrowed arteries weakens the heart and arteries, impedes blood flow to vital organs such as the kidneys, brain and eyes, and predisposes to heart attacks and strokes. The most common causes of high blood pressure are hereditary tendency, stress, obesity, kidney problems, excess alcohol and smoking and hardening of the arteries.

Treatment
The best antihypertensive herbs that relax and dilate arteries include Hawthorn, Lime flower, Garlic, Gingko, Motherwort, Cramp bark, Valerian and Gotu kola. Antioxidant herbs Amalaki, Holy basil, Selfheal, Turmeric, Shiitake mushroom, Blueberry/ Bilberry, Elderberry, Ginger, Red grape seed extract and Guggulu prevent damage to arteries from free radicals and reduce the risk of heart attacks and strokes.

For problems related to anxiety and tension, you could add to your prescription Cramp bark, Rosemary, Wild oats, Chamomile or Passion flower. Lime flower tea is relaxing and dilates the arteries, reducing blood pressure.

For excess fluid, take diuretic herbs such as Dandelion leaves, Corn silk, Cleavers or Goldenrod.

Other measures
A predominantly vegetarian diet and use of cold-pressed vegetable oils are recommended. You should avoid tea, coffee, alcohol and smoking, and take regular aerobic exercise. Meditation and yoga sessions can also be very helpful.

Caution
Seek medical attention if you suffer from high blood pressure.

RAISED CHOLESTEROL

There are two types of cholesterol. The first is low-density lipoproteins (LDL), which increase the risk of heart attacks. The second is high-density lipoproteins (HDL), which actually reduce the risk of heart attacks. Cholesterol is a fatty, waxy substance, 25 per cent of which comes from food and the rest is manufactured in the liver. Excess sugar, refined carbohydrates and fats and errors of liver metabolism are largely to blame for high LDL.

Treatment
Antioxidant herbs including Hawthorn, Cayenne pepper, Red grape seed extract, Guggulu, Blueberry/Bilberry, Elderberry, Ginger, Evening primrose, Chinese angelica and Liquorice protect arteries, inhibit formation of atherosclerotic plaque, lower cholesterol and help prevent cardiovascular disease.

Shiitake and Reishi mushrooms and Wild oats contain beta-glucans, which help lower cholesterol. A garlic clove a day can substantially lower cholesterol levels, and Red clover reduces its absorption.

Other measures
Niacin (vitamin B3) lowers total cholesterol as well as LDL cholesterol, triglycerides and fibrinogen, a blood protein responsible for forming clots. It also raises HDL. Take in a B-complex supplement. Reduce high-fat foods, red meats and fried foods. Replace saturated oils with monosaturated ones like Olive and Avocado oils and polyunsaturated fats as in nuts, seeds, Flax seed and fish oils. Plant fibres can lower cholesterol, so a diet high in fruit and vegetables and whole grains with minimal fats helps maintain normal cholesterol levels. Take regular aerobic exercise.

HERBS FOR THE MUSCULOSKELETAL SYSTEM

The health of our musculoskeletal system depends on good diet and efficient digestion, absorption and elimination. Overusing or neglecting certain groups of muscles, posture and the amount of fresh air and exercise we take all have their effect. Stress and the inability to relax put a strain on the system and can contribute to joint and muscle problems, but the biggest factor is age. From around the age of 30 our bone density diminishes and accelerates in women after the menopause, meaning that our bones become more fragile and prone to fractures and breaks. Horsetail and Comfrey nourish the bones, Aloe vera, Wild celery seed, Burdock, Devil's claw and Liquorice help prevent and remedy joint problems, while Cramp bark, Rosemary, Hops and St John's wort help to relax tense muscles and prevent them from damage.

ARTHRITIS

Arthritis causes joint stiffness and inflammation, and can lead to degeneration of the joints, disfigurement and pain. Osteoarthritis involving wear and tear is most common; rheumatoid arthritis is a more serious and progressive autoimmune disease. Underlying causes include poor diet, digestive problems, dysbiosis, toxicity, free radical damage, age, stress and chronic infection. Poor digestion and constipation cause nutritional deficiency and accumulation of toxins in the gut, which are absorbed into the circulation and contribute to joint problems.

Treatment

Turmeric and Frankincense can be used for osteoarthritis and rheumatoid arthritis, as they are potent antioxidants, enhance immunity, reduce pain and inflammation and have an affinity with muscles and bones. Devil's claw and Myrrh are excellent anti-inflammatories that reduce pain and stiffness. Black cohosh is anti-inflammatory and analgesic, excellent for post-menopausal arthritis. Liquorice has cortisone-like anti-inflammatory actions and increases tolerance to physical and emotional stress. Ashwagandha, with its painkilling and anti-inflammatory action and immunostimulating properties, is ideal for autoimmune problems like rheumatoid arthritis. Long pepper, Turmeric and Cinnamon improve digestion, while Burdock, Nettle, Yellow dock, Marigold and Cleavers clear toxins. Other beneficial herbs include Meadowsweet, Bladderwrack, Gotu kola, Shiitake mushroom, Echinacea, Wild yam, Feverfew, Willow and Angelica.

Take Ginger tea daily as an anti-inflammatory and antioxidant to reduce pain and swelling and the associated bursitis.

Massage using liniments that contain essential oils of Rosemary, Peppermint, Lavender or Sweet marjoram with a few drops of Cayenne pepper tincture will increase circulation to the joints and decrease pain.

Other measures
Supplements of Evening primrose oil, glucosamine sulphate, methylsulfonylmethane (MSM), Rose hip, omega-3 oils and selenium all protect and promote the repair of cartilage.

GOUT

Gout is caused by a build-up of uric acid in the blood. Uric acid is a by-product of protein metabolism in the liver, and when this reaches a certain level, uric acid crystals form and collect in joints, causing intense pain, swelling and inflammation. It usually starts in the big toe first. It tends to run in families, is more common in men who are overweight and associated with high blood pressure and triglycerides.

Treatment
Diuretics, especially Wild celery seed and Nettle, but also Gravel root, Fennel, Wild oat straw, Cleavers or Goldenrod help the kidneys eliminate excess uric acid and other toxins. You can combine these with anti-inflammatory Devil's claw, Turmeric, Liquorice, Cat's claw, Rose hip,

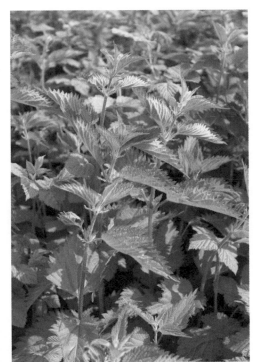

Nettles have been shown in studies to relieve the pain of arthritis.

Olive leaf, Willow, Meadowsweet, Frankincense, Ginger, Sarsaparilla or Wild yam to reduce joint pain and swelling, along with herbs to support the liver such as Burdock, Gentian, Milk thistle or Rosemary.

Externally painful joints can be massaged with essential oils of Peppermint, Rosemary or Lavender oil in sesame oil.

Other measures

Gout is related to excess fatty foods, purines (from red meat, organ meats and shellfish), nightshades (potatoes, peppers, aubergines and tomatoes), cheese, citrus fruits and alcohol (particularly beer), so adjust your diet accordingly. It can also be triggered by certain drugs, crash diets and exercise, therefore take pre-emptive action. Bromelain from pineapple is excellent for acute attacks and can be taken as a supplement along with quercitrin and vitamin C from cherries to prevent future attacks.

OSTEOPOROSIS

Loss of bone tissue actually begins in our 30s, but is hastened through lower oestrogen levels after the menopause. Other contributing factors are poor digestion and absorption, lack of calcium and other important bone nutrients including essential fatty acids, vitamin D, magnesium and boron in the diet, smoking, lack of exercise and a

history of total hysterectomy. Women who are underweight, who have dieted frequently or suffered from coeliac disease are more at risk, as oestrogen is stored in fat tissue. It is indicated by a tendency to fractures, back pain, loss of height due to compression of the spine and muscle spasm.

Treatment

Use oestrogenic herbs like Shatavari, Chinese angelica, Red clover, Marigold, Wild yam, Liquorice, Sage, Hops or Siberian ginseng, combined with herbs to improve digestion and absorption, including Long pepper, Ginger, Fennel or Coriander.

Evening primrose oil or Borage seed oil will help hormone balance.

Calcium-rich herbs are also important such as Nettle, Dandelion leaf, Horsetail, Bladderwrack, Dill, Wild celery seed, Wild oats, Borage, Codonopsis, Hawthorn and Amalaki.

Other measures

Plenty of exercise and supplements of vitamins E and D, magnesium and boron are recommended.

MUSCLE PAIN AND FIBROMYALGIA

Tender, stiff and aching muscles can occur after unaccustomed exercise, while more extreme muscle pain is caused by cramp, muscle strain or other injuries such as a compressed nerve; the muscles affected or those nearby can go into spasm, which further increases the pain. If muscle tension or spasm is prolonged, tender lumps, which are fibrositic nodules, may develop. Generalized muscle pain combined with fatigue and malaise can be a symptom of chronic stress, overwork, tiredness, flu and fibromyalgia (which is associated with post-viral fatigue syndrome).

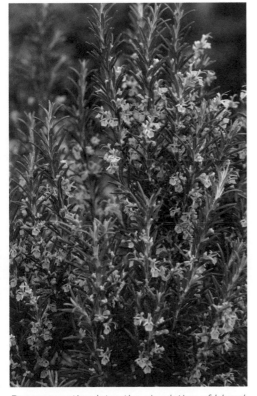

Rosemary stimulates the circulation of blood and has a restorative effect on both the body and the mind.

Treatment

Massage tense and aching muscles with essential oils of Rosemary, Thyme, Holy basil, Lavender, Chamomile or Ginger diluted in sesame oil. This will increase circulation to the affected area, ease tension and spasm and reduce pain. Sesame oil is rich in calcium and magnesium, which help release muscle tension. Muscle-relaxing herbs Rosemary, Thyme, Chamomile, Ginger, Lavender, Holy basil, Black cohosh, Wild yam and Ashwagandha can be taken internally; the latter has a special affinity with muscle tissue.

For inflammation after an injury or muscle strain, use anti-inflammatory Frankincense, Devil's claw, Liquorice, Meadowsweet, Ginger, Black willow, Turmeric, Black cohosh or Cat's claw.

Adaptogenic, immune-enhancing and tonic herbs such as Ashwagandha, Siberian ginseng and Shiitake mushroom are helpful for states of depletion and fibromyalgia.

Other measures

Rest aching muscles if they develop from overuse, but only for 2–3 days, after which gently start to stretch them. Supplements of calcium and magnesium can help to reduce muscle pain and spasm.

MAINTAINING HEALTHY SKIN

To keep your skin healthy, eat a well-balanced diet that includes plenty of protein, essential fatty acids, particularly omega-3s from oily fish and flax seeds, and antioxidants from fresh organic fruit and vegetables.

Deficiencies of minerals, vitamins and trace elements and excess junk foods that create toxicity can impair the skin's resilience and predispose it to a number of disorders. Herbs can increase blood flow to the skin, providing vital nutrients and helping clear toxins.

ECZEMA

Eczema is a systemic problem, not simply an external irritation. An allergic reaction to foods such as wheat, gluten or dairy foods or other external irritants such as animal dander and house dust mites is often involved. The local immune mechanisms in the skin may be put under pressure by underuse of the other eliminative pathways, the bowels and kidneys, or immunity may be lowered by dietary deficiencies, chronic toxicity, poor digestion, dysbiosis and stress. Adverse drug reactions and irritants such as washing powder can also be implicated.

Treatment

To soothe the allergic response, use antihistamines Chamomile, Yarrow, Feverfew, Nettle,

Baikal skullcap or Lemon balm. Adaptogenic herbs Ashwagandha, Guduchi, Amalaki, Schisandra, Liquorice, Shiitake and Reishi mushrooms, Aloe vera and Ginseng increase general immunity and improve resilience to stress. Gentle relaxants Chamomile, Passion flower, Vervain, Lavender and Rosemary reduce tension and anxiety.

Cleansing herbs support the liver's detoxifying work, taking the strain off the skin. Burdock, Red clover, Cleavers, Nettle, Neem, Dandelion, Globe artichoke, Milk thistle and Aloe vera clear heat and inflammation.

Creams or oils containing Chamomile, Evening primrose oil, Marigold, Chickweed, Comfrey, Lavender, or Aloe vera gel, can soothe inflammation. Evening primrose oil or Borage seed oil will provide gamma-linolenic acid (GLA), often deficient in eczema.

Other measures
Vitamins A, B, C and E, zinc magnesium, calcium and iron are also considered essential.

ACNE

Overactive sebaceous glands due in part to hormonal changes especially during adolescence make

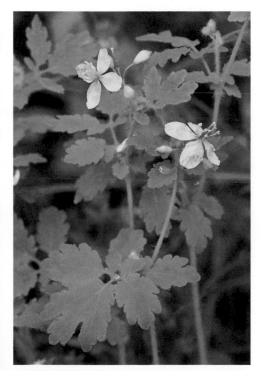

Greater celandine is a herb that encourages the skin to heal.

the skin oily. The sebum blocks hair follicles, causing them to become inflamed and infected, producing the characteristic blackheads and spots. Acne is also indicative of nutritional deficiencies, toxicity, dysbiosis, stressed adrenals, PCOS and certain food allergies.

Treatment
It is important to support the liver and bowels in their detoxifying work to take the load off the skin as an eliminative organ and prevent a build-up of hormones in the body. Use Burdock, Milk thistle, Dandelion root, Red clover, Guduchi, Cleavers, Liquorice or Yellow dock. For constipation, take 1–2 teaspoons of Linseeds or Psyllium seeds soaked in a little warm water before bed.

To clear the skin, use antimicrobial and anti-inflammatory herbs like Echinacea, Neem, Myrrh, Turmeric, Amalaki, Oregon grape and Wild indigo. Other cleansing herbs include Nettle, Bhringaraj, Borage, Aloe vera, Pau d'arco, Cat's claw, Wild pansy and Andrographis Hormone. Balancing herbs include Chaste tree, Wild yam, Evening primrose oil and Saw palmetto.

Leave the skin alone; clean it daily with Rose water, apply infusions of Marigold, Elderflower or Lavender afterwards and never squeeze pimples. Once the skin has cleared, use a few drops of either Neroli or Lavender oil in aqueous cream,

Comfrey or vitamin E cream, to heal the scars.

Other measures
Avoid fatty foods, dairy produce, chocolate, alcohol, sweets, red meats, iodine-rich foods, tea and coffee.

PSORIASIS

A complex autoimmune skin problem, psoriasis speeds up the normal growth and renewal of skin cells by five to ten times and produces the build-up of scaly patches that can appear almost anywhere on the body. It can affect fingernails, leaving them discoloured, pitted or split, and is sometimes associated with polyarthritis. It may be hereditary or triggered by excess alcohol, sunburn, skin injury, a streptococcal throat infection, stress or shock, and can be improved by sunlight and visits to the Dead Sea. Food allergies, incomplete protein digestion, dysbiosis, poor liver function and nutritional deficiencies can also play a part.

Treatment
Herbs containing psoralens such as Angelica, Wild carrot, Wild celery seed and Fennel help clear the

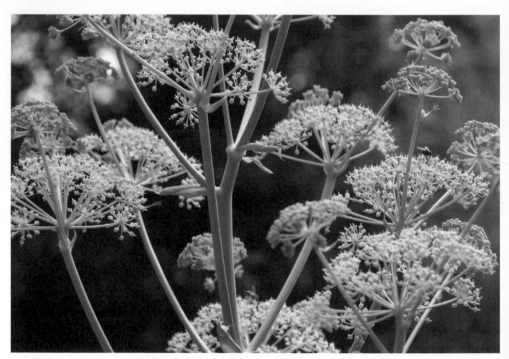

Fennel has a clarifying effect on skin conditions and is an anti-inflammatory herb.

skin, especially in combination with sunbathing. Antioxidant herbs like Oregon grape, Barberry, Golden seal or Red grape seed extract reduce free radical damage to the skin and decrease inflammation. Alkaloids in Oregon grape root slow proliferation of skin cells. Milk thistle and Forskohlii can also slow down the growth of skin cells. Sarsaparilla, Honeysuckle, Frankincense, raw Rehmannia root, Neem, Turmeric, Evening primrose oil and Peony are other good anti-inflammatories.

To aid the liver in its detoxifying work, use Burdock, Yellow dock, Red clover, Turmeric or Dandelion. Guggulu is also excellent.

Externally, creams containing Chamomile, Liquorice, Turmeric, Lavender oil, Evening primrose oil, Aloe vera juice, Oregon grape, capsaicin from Cayenne pepper or Wild oats can help clear the skin.

Other measures
Supplements of omega-3 essential fatty acids, vitamin A and zinc are recommended.

MOUTH AND GUM PROBLEMS

Good oral hygiene and a healthy immune system will generally keep at bay infections that can develop from the many micro-organisms that generally inhabit the mouth. Lowered immunity from poor diet, chronic illness such as diabetes, digestive problems, dysbiosis, food allergies, alcohol, smoking, stress, tiredness and mercury fillings can predispose to infections and inflammatory problems, including bleeding gums and mouth ulcers.

Treatment
Antimicrobial and anti-inflammatory herbs such as Echinacea, Cat's claw, Myrrh, Sage, Thyme, Marigold, Chamomile, Golden seal or Peppermint can be used as mouthwashes to combat infections in the mouth and taken internally to improve immunity and to remedy gut problems and dysbiosis. Bitter, detoxifying herbs Burdock, Dandelion, Milk thistle, Guduchi, Amalaki or Yellow dock can be added to support the work of the liver.

Astringent herbs like Plantain, Thyme, Marigold, Agrimony, Rose, Vervain, Periwinkle and Yarrow make good mouthwashes for strengthening gums and stopping bleeding, while antioxidants taken internally, such as Guduchi, Blueberry/Bilberry, Hawthorn, Cat's claw, Selfheal, Common grape vine and Sweet marjoram, will help to protect blood vessels from free radical damage.

Other measures
As preventative measures, it is important to floss regularly and rinse the mouth daily with herbal antiseptics.

HERBS FOR THE EYES

Certain nutrients are vital to eye health. Elderberries and Blueberries/Bilberries are rich in antioxidant anthocyanosides, which contain or boost the action of gluthione an antioxidant in the acqueous humour, helping prevent cataracts. Anthocyanidins protect blood vessels in the eye, preventing poor night vision and retinal disorders.

CONJUNCTIVITIS AND STYES

In conjunctivitis the lining of the eye becomes irritated either by infection, allergy such as hay fever and rhinitis, dust or pollution in the atmosphere, and the eye becomes red and inflamed, often weepy. Styes result from inflammation or infections of the glands at the base of the eyelashes and tend to occur when run-down or tired.

Treatment
To soothe irritated and inflamed eyes, infusions of astringent and antiseptic herbs Eyebright, Marigold, Chamomile, Elderflower and Rose can be taken internally and used to bathe the eyes. Black tea is a useful remedy to bathe the eyes, or lay a warm Chamomile tea bag over each eye and leave in place for 10–15 minutes. Apply warm infusions of Eyebright, Chamomile, Elderflower, Plantain or Marigold as compresses.

For chronic conjunctivitis, take supplements of Borage seed oil or Evening primrose oil.

Caution
Use a sterilized eyebath and don't use the same solution for both eyes.

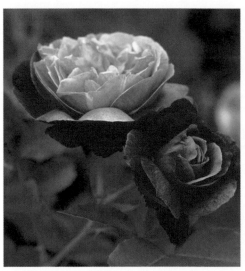

Rose, prepared as an infusion, makes a soothing eyebath for sore or inflamed eyes.

HERBS AND THE HORMONAL SYSTEM

Many herbs are beneficial to the hormonal system. Liquorice and Echinacea support the thymus gland in its immune work; Bladderwrack and Ashwagandha influence the thyroid; Chaste tree helps to regulate the pituitary gland; Liquorice, Wild yam, Ginseng and Borage influence the adrenals; Wild yam, Black cohosh, Chaste tree, Shatavari, Ashwagandha and Ginseng all help regulate reproductive hormones. Bitter herbs such as Dandelion root, Milk thistle and Burdock aid the liver's breakdown of hormones so that they are excreted from the body once they have done their work.

PREMENSTRUAL SYNDROME (PMS)

The familiar physical, mental and emotional symptoms of PMS in the second half of the cycle are generally linked to excess oestrogen in relation to progesterone. Environmental toxins from plastics, polychlorinated biphenyls (PCBs) and pesticides that mimic oestrogen in the body as well as oestrogen residues in tap water and meat, and the liver's inability to break down oestrogen, disrupt normal hormone balance.

Treatment

Chaste tree is the best-known herb to increase progesterone and is generally taken as tincture, ½ teaspoon 30 minutes before breakfast. Adaptogenic herbs Wild yam, Liquorice, Ashwagandha, Shatavari, Chinese angelica and Black cohosh, are rich in steroidal saponins and increase resilience to stress and balance hormones. Nervines help to stabilize emotions and include Wild oats, Chamomile, Gotu kola, Bhringaraj and Motherwort.

Liver herbs such as Burdock, Dandelion, Guduchi, Milk thistle, Barberry and Yellow dock are important to help the breakdown of hormones.

Diuretic herbs Cleavers, Dandelion, Corn silk, Fennel, Coriander, Wild celery and Wild carrot help relieve fluid retention, bloating and breast discomfort.

A supplement of Evening primrose oil is also recommended for easing PMS symptoms.

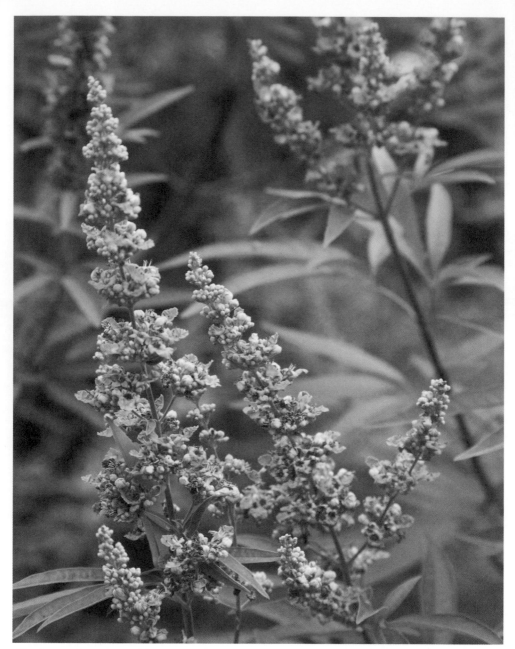

Chaste tree is renowned for its ability to balance hormones through its action on the pituitary gland.

MENSTRUAL PROBLEMS

These are largely due to hormone imbalances and nutritional deficiencies. Irregular or absent periods are associated with intense exercise, nutritional deficiency, sudden weight loss, drugs and psychological stress or shock. Other endocrine disorders can be involved.

Painful periods are related to poor circulation, stress, overwork and muscular tension, lack of exercise, bad posture and caffeine. Heavy periods can be caused by fibroids, polyps, thyroid problems, uterine congestion and perimenopause.

Treatment

To regulate hormones, use Chaste tree, Wild yam, Chinese angelica or Shatavari with Liquorice and Evening primrose oil. You can combine these with liver herbs like Burdock, Holy thistle, Oregon grape or Dandelion to aid the breakdown of hormones.

For intense cramps with scanty bleeding, Cramp bark, Black haw, Motherwort, Pasque flower and Black cohosh are excellent taken every two hours when necessary. For associated tension, add Valerian, Passion flower, Chamomile or Hops. The rubbing oils of Chamomile, Lavender or Rosemary gently into the abdomen will help relieve pain.

For heavy bleeding, astringent herbs such as Beth root, Yarrow, Periwinkle, Lady's mantle, Agrimony, Chinese Foxglove, Bayberry and Rose can be taken three to six times daily.

Iron-containing foods and herbs, such as Nettle, Coriander leaf, Codonopsis, Amalaki, Bladderwrack and Yellow dock, help combat anaemia.

Other measures

Avoid caffeine, alcohol and refined and junk foods, and take supplements of vitamins B-complex and C, as well as zinc and magnesium. Also take regular exercise.

VAGINAL INFECTIONS

The delicate environment of pH and flora of the vagina can be disturbed by hormonal imbalances, antibiotics, stress, poor diet, the contraceptive pill, pregnancy, post-menopausal changes and diabetes, and become susceptible to inflammation and infection. Yeast infections (thrush) are most common and tend to be related to gut dysbiosis. Trichomonas, gardnerella, human papillomavirus (HPV), or vaginal warts, herpes and bacterial vaginiosis (common after the menopause) can also occur.

Treatment

Antiseptic herbs to combat infection include Marigold, Golden seal, Thyme, Chamomile, Lavender, Pau d'arco, Neem, Turmeric, Echinacea and Sweet marjoram, which can be taken internally and used in creams,

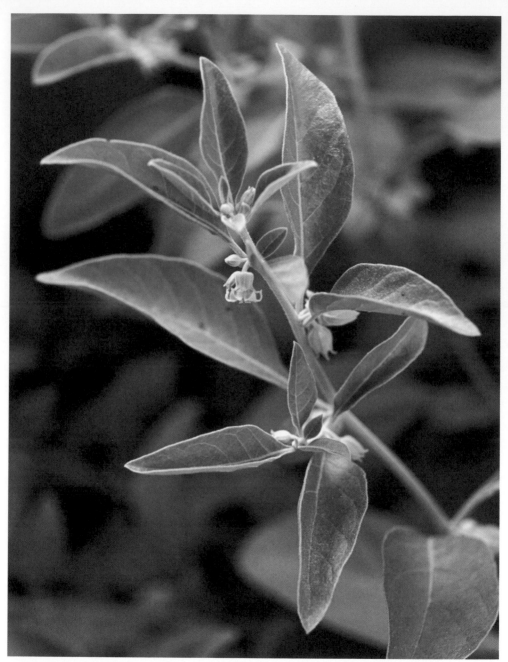

Ashwagandha enhances resilience to stress and has a balancing effect on the hormones.

douches, and in lotions in which tampons can be soaked and inserted for 30 minutes morning and night.

Garlic is a great antimicrobial for internal and external use, active against bacterial, viral and fungal infections like thrush. Peel a clove carefully without nicking it, wrap it in clean gauze and insert for 6 consecutive nights. Alternatively, add 5 ml (1 teaspoon) of fresh garlic juice to a few tablespoons of live yogurt, soak a tampon in it or use as a douche twice daily. If the area is sore and inflamed, sitting in a bowl of Chamomile tea is relieving.

The above herbs will resolve infection in the vagina and more systemic problems of toxicity and dysbiosis. Immune-enhancing herbs like Ashwagandha, Shatavari, Guduchi, Amalaki and Schisandra can be taken following an infection to prevent further problems.

Caution
Seek medical attention if you suspect sexually transmitted infection.

MENOPAUSAL PROBLEMS

Low libido, hot flushes, night sweats, mood swings, 'mid-life crises', depression and insomnia are some of the symptoms that can characterize the menopause, when levels of oestrogen and progesterone decline to the point where menstruation ceases. The adrenal glands take over production of similar hormones, but stress and adrenal exhaustion can impair their ability to do so adequately, triggering the familiar symptoms. Subsequent health problems include increased risk of osteoporosis and heart and arterial disease.

Treatment
Several plants contain isoflavones, similar in structure to oestrogen, called phytoestrogens. They occur in Shatavari, Red clover, Chinese angelica, Wild yam, Wild indigo, Siberian ginseng, Liquorice and Black cohosh. These herbs also support the adrenals, increase resilience to stress and are very helpful for relieving menopausal symptoms.

Chaste tree, Motherwort, Sage, Chamomile, Hops, Lady's mantle, Aloe vera, Hawthorn, Fennel, Sarsaparilla and Rehmannia will also reduce menopausal symptoms. Burdock, Dandelion, Holy thistle and Milk thistle aid the liver's metabolism of hormones, while relaxants Chamomile, Pasque flower, Motherwort, Vervain, Wild oats and Lemon balm are calming where anxiety is aggravating symptoms.

Supplements of Borage seed oil or Evening primrose oil are also helpful.

Other measures
Supplements of vitamin E, calcium and magnesium are recommended.

LOW SEX DRIVE/IMPOTENCE

Lack of sexual interest in men and women and erectile dysfunction in men are increasingly common problems. Hormone imbalances, stress, depression, pain, obesity, poor health, low energy, marital problems, diabetes, high blood pressure, circulatory problems and the effects of drugs and smoking are all contributory factors.

Treatment

Herbs for balancing hormones and increasing sexual energy include Ashwagandha, Shatavari, Chinese angelica, Liquorice ,Schisandra and Korean and Siberian ginseng. These adaptogenic remedies also increase resilience to stress and counter the effects of anxiety and depression.

Wild oats, Rose, Rosemary, Gotu kola and Vervain are all considered to be good relaxants.

Black cohosh, Wild yam, Sage, Motherwort and Chaste tree balance hormones during the menopause, while Sarsaparilla and Saw palmetto all support the production of male hormones. Gingko, Ginger, Hawthorn and Gotu kola can help circulatory problems.

Detoxifying remedies including Burdock, Nettle, Yellow dock and Milk thistle can be taken to support the liver and clear the side effects of drugs.

INFERTILITY AND LOW SPERM COUNT

Infertility is reaching epidemic proportions, related largely to the effect of environmental toxins and residues of the contraceptive pill in water supplies, which are causing widespread hormonal imbalances. Hernia surgery, tubule infection, chlamydia, diabetes, drugs, mumps, stress, smoking, toxic metals and nutritional deficiencies may all affect sperm count.

Treatment

Detoxifying herbs such as Bladderwrack, Burdock, Andrographis, Globe artichoke, Shiitake and Reishi mushrooms, Guduchi, Milk thistle and Nettle can be taken to support the liver's breakdown of drugs and toxins.

Hormone-balancing and adaptogenic herbs to enhance fertility are Ashwagandha, Shatavari, Chaste tree, Wild yam, Chinese angelica, Schisandra, Liquorice and Korean and Siberian ginseng. They also increase resilience to stress and counter the effects of anxiety and depression.

Black cohosh, Motherwort, Evening primrose oil and Rose can also be used for menstrual problems.

Other measures

Supplements of vitamins B-complex and E, zinc, omega-3 and -6 oils and coenzyme Q10 are recommended.

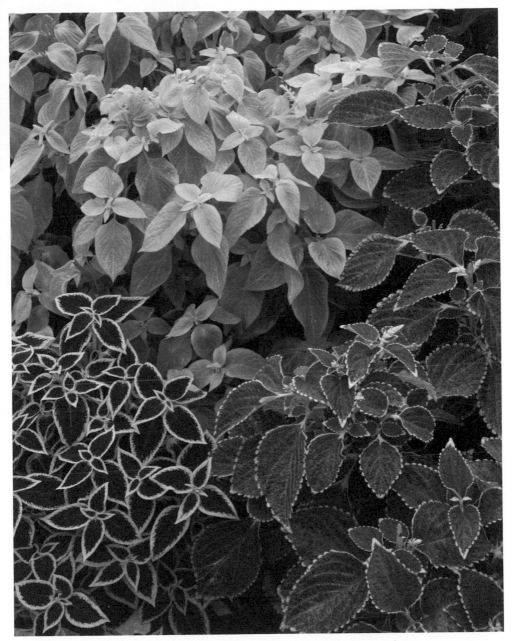

Forskkohlii contains forskolin, which stimulates the release of hormones from the thyroid gland.

Pesticides are designed to disrupt the reproductive cycle of the insect, fungus or weed it is trying to kill, so eat organic produce.

THYROID PROBLEMS

The thyroid gland works in conjunction with the pituitary gland, which produces thyroid-stimulating hormone (TSH) to make the hormones T3 and T4, which play a vital role in metabolism. Hypothyroidism, when the thyroid is underactive, is more common after menopause and causes slow metabolism, low energy, weight gain, fluid retention and dry skin and hair. Hyperthyroidism, when it is overactive (commonly related to autoimmune disease as in Hashimoto's disease, or to a cyst on the thyroid) causes goitre, weight loss, anxiety, heat intolerance and palpitations. Thyroid imbalances are complex and linked to poor diet, excess sugar, stress, adrenal exhaustion, hormonal changes, viruses, environmental toxins, food allergies and dysbiosis.

Treatment Forskohlii, Guggulu and Bladderwrack increase the production of thyroid hormones and regulate the thyroid. For autoimmune problems, detoxifying herbs that help metabolism include Oregon grape, Dandelion root, Gentian, Yellow dock, Horsetail and Barberry. They can be combined with adaptogens Ashwagandha, Bacopa, Gotu kola, Wild oats, Polygonum and Siberian ginseng, which are high in antioxidants, to regulate thyroid activity, enhance immunity and increase resilience to stress. To calm an overactive thyroid, try Meadowsweet, Motherwort and Lemon balm.

Other measures

Supplements of selenium, zinc and vitamin E and B6 help conversion of T4 to T3.

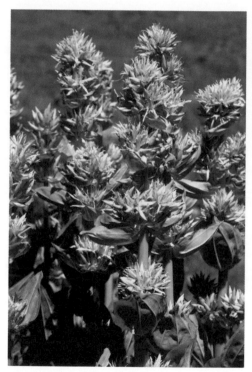

Gentian is a detoxifying herb. It helps the metabolism and can be useful for autoimmune problems.

INDEX

ACKNOWLEDGEMENTS

Material previously published as *The Gaia Complete Herbal Tutor* in 2010 by Gaia, a division of Octopus Publishing Group Ltd

Special Photography:
© **Octopus Publishing Group**/Ruth Jenkinson

Other Photography:
Alamy/Peter Arnold, Inc. 168; /blickwinkel 143; /Adrian Davies 129; /Bob Gibbons 161; /Steffen Hauser/botanikfoto 139; /kpzfoto 136; /McPhoto 172. **Private Collection**/The Stapleton Collection 6. **ChinaFotoPress** 10. **Corbis**/Envision 130; /Gerd Ludwig 13. **Fotolia**/adisa 141; /Martina Berg 137; /Alison Bowden 17; /Olga Shelego 2, 126; /jerome whittingham 157. **Octopus Publishing Group**/Michael Boyes 123; /William Lingwood 27; /Russell Sadur 29; /David Sarton. **Photolibrary**/Gerrit Buntrock 152; /Pablo Galan Cela 141; /Georgianna Lane 148; /Andrea Jones 144; /Antonio Molero 135; /Pixtal Images 133; /Isabelle Plasschaert 15; /Radius Images 16; /Howard Rice 164; /Mark Turner 18, 151, 166. **Wellcome Library, London** 23.